Rewired FOR Sleep

THE 28-DAY INSOMNIA REPAIR MANUAL

Daniel R. Bernstein, L. Ac., CH

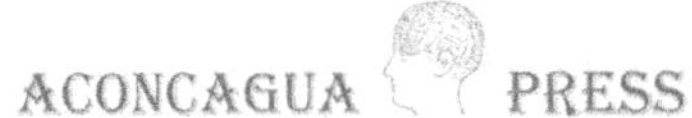

ACONCAGUA PRESS

REWIRED FOR SLEEP

Copyright

Disclaimer

This book is designed to help you understand how you may use your innate abilities to sleep through the night by making informed lifestyle choices.

The publication contains the opinions and ideas of its author. It is intended to provide helpful and informative material on the subjects addressed in the publication.

It is sold with the understanding that the author and Aconcagua Press are not engaged in rendering medical, health, or any other kind of personal professional services in this book. The reader should consult his or her medical, health, or other licensed physician before adopting any of the suggestions in this book or drawing inferences from it.

The author and Aconcagua Press specifically disclaim all responsibility for any liability, loss or damage, personal or otherwise, which may be incurred or alleged to have been incurred directly or indirectly by the use and application of any of the information contained in this book.

Dedication

Dedicated with gratitude and affection to my patients, whose personal struggles, and triumphs, helped form the strategies and templates that make up the guts and soul of this book.

TABLE OF CONTENTS

Copyright i

Disclaimer i

Dedication v

TABLE OF CONTENTS vii

Acknowledgements 17

Preface xix

Introduction xxvii

PART I: 33

Sleeping in the Material World 33

Chapter 1: Insomniac's Guide to the Underworld 1

A Map of the Map 1

Exercise 1: The V-A-K Sensor 2

The Power of Touch 4

The Power of Words 4

Exercise 2: My Friend John/Jane 5

Sleep Journal 7

Chapter 2: Under Pressure: The Cop and the Restless Leg 3

Acupressure for Sleep 5

Exercise 3: The Five, Five, and Five 6

Chapter 3: The Barriers to Sleep, & Sleep Hygiene 9

The Barriers to Sleep 9

Sleep Hygiene 10

Daniel's Extended Sleep Hygiene List 14

Removing More Barriers to Sleep 16

Chapter 4 Stress and Lifestyle 21

David and the Spaghetti-Tangled Mind 21

Lifestyle 23

Breathe! (Abdominal Breathing) 24

Exercise 4: Move the Voice (V-A) 26

Exercise 5: Remake Your Day 27

Break-in: Under 3rd Toe 30

Chapter 5 Case of the Runaway Bride (Meridian Tapping) 33

Exercise 6: Meridian Tapping 34

Darrell Taps on Anger 40

Chapter 6: Progressive Muscle Relaxation............................45

Luis and Rebound Insomnia 45

Relax the Muscles, Relax the Mind 47

Exercise 7: Progressive Muscle Relaxation........................47

*Bonus point: Gallbladder 30. 50

Chapter 7: The Case for the Elastic Brain 51

The Pauli Exclusion Principle..51

Neuroplasticity...53

Exercise 8: Autogenic Training 54

Exercise 9: Use Your Words About Sleep Wisely.................57

Affirmations, and the Power of Words 58

Chapter 8: Chinese Medicine, and Ancient Tattoos 63

Ötzi Gets Some Ink........................63

The Inner Thermostat........................64

Chapter 9: How I Learned to Stop Worrying and Love Qi Gong 69

Hearing the Voice Within. 69

Exercise 10: Six Healing Sounds (Liu Zi Jue)........................70

Liver/Gallbladder (helps control the quality of the blood and supports eyesight)........................71

Heart/Small Intestine........................73

Spleen/Stomach/Pancreas (controls transportation of nutrients) 74

Lungs/Large Intestine (controls the intake of oxygen)....75

Kidneys/Bladder 76

Triple Warmer/Pericardium (harmonizes all the organs) 77

Chapter 10: Nutrition Impossible? Sleep-Positive Food 81

Sleep-Positive Food 81

Specific Foods That Encourage Sleep........................82

Food to Avoid........................83

Amino Acids That Support Sleep 86

Food for Thought: Acknowledge the Voice........................88

Chapter 11: Ear-Shaped Box: Auriculotherapy........................91

Your Inner Toolkit........................91

Auriculotherapy Tools: 93

Tiger Warmers, Heat Therapy 95

.Chapter 12: The Question of Sleep Aids 99

"To Dose, Or Not to Dose" 99

Benzodiazepines and the "Z" Drugs: A Primer 99

The "Z" Drugs 100

The Facts About Medication 101

Sleep-aids: What Exactly Do They Do? 102

The Stages of Sleep 102

Stage One: Drifting Off: 102

Stage Two: Sinking Deeper: 103

Stage Three: Deep Sleep 103

Stage Four: REM Sleep: 103

Are Sleep Aids Restorative? 103

Who is to Blame for Our "Sleep Aid" Problem? 104

Heart 7: Spirit Gate 105

Pericardium 6: Inner Pass 106

Chapter 13: In Her Mind, She Left it All Behind 109

Dina Hangs Her Problems on a Hook 109

Dina Creates a Model for Tranquility 111

Exercise 11: The Butterfly Hug 114

Exercise 12: Staircase to Your Special Place (V-K) 115

Chapter 14: Herbal Options 119

Sleep-Positive Herbs 119

Western Herbs 120

Hops (Humulus lupulus): 120

Valerian (Valeriana officinalis) : 120

Kava (Piper methysticum): 120

Chamomile: 120

Passionflower (Passiflora): 121

CBD (Cannabidiol): 121

St. John's Wort (Hypericum perforate): 121

California Poppy : 121

Cordyceps Sinensis: 122

Western Herbal Formulas for Insomnia 122

Herbal Break-In: Turmeri-Cola!..................................123

Chapter 15: Unplug from Anxiety................................127

Anxiety, Sleep Killer #1 127

Exercise 13: Four-Step Trauma Intervention (FSTI).......128

Jenna Reclaims Her Brain (Prefrontal Cortex Anxiety) 131

Jenna does Four-Step Trauma Intervention....................131

Chapter 16: Fatigue, and Refilling the Empty Well 137

Michelle Hits the Wall..137

Adrenal Fatigue 138

Adrenal Repair 139

Exercise 14: The Reverse Spin 140

Bonus Ear Protocol: Stress 144

Chapter 17: Reclaiming Control of the Mind 147

When the Sleep Wagon Is Wobbly 147

Erika 148

What Is Trance (aka self-hypnosis, or guided visualization)? 149

History of Trance 149

Trance Today 150

Method I: 151

Exercise 15: The Betty E. Self-Hypnosis Method 151

Getting Started 152

Affirmations on Sleep: 152

Entering into Self-Trance (V-A-K) 153

Part I (The External Section) 153

Part II: The Internal Section 154

Chapter 18: Barbara is a Punk Wiccan (Paradoxical Insomnia) 157

My Friend John/Jane 158

What are Essential Oils? 159

PART II 167

Perchance to Sleep: 167

Rewiring the Circuits 167

Helene: Phoenix Rises from the Ashes, and Flies 170

Jeffrey Runs PTSD Down (Maintenance Insomnia) 176

Auricular PTSD Protocol 177

Short Form Tapping 179

Exercise 16: Desensitize Touch Protocol for Pain 180

Case of The Sleep-Disturbed Leopard (Onset Insomnia) 182

Annabelle and the Reverse Spin 183

Kava's Fine, but 185

Ginger Rogers and the Hot Flash 188

Phytoestrogen Rich Food 190

Raymond's Path: Detoxing from Sleep Aids 190

Weaning Yourself Off Medication 191

Tools for Detoxification. 192

The Rewired Detox Program 195

Pediatric Acupressure 196

PART III 201

Journey to the Center 201

The Extra Mile 1.5 203

Meditation 203

Inner Smile Part I 204

Microcosmic Orbit 206

Inner Smile II 208

Autogenic Training, Part II 210

The 7-Day Neuroplasticity Challenge 211

Change Things Up (a V-A-K Trifecta) 212

Meridian Tapping II: Other Voices, Other Modules 213

Drug Detoxification: 214

Guided Meditation: Your Special Place 217

The Beach 218

The Garden Path 218

Honduran Rainforest (Heart-Centered Meditation) 219

The Lake 220

The 28-Day Insomnia Repair Program 223

Week Three: Quick Change Artist, or the 7-Day Challenge
.... 231

Week Four: Magical Mystery Microcosmic Orbit 235

Glossary of Acupoints and Their Functions 241

Bibliography 247

Books You May Find Interesting 251

About the Author 253

THE REWIRED SANCTUARY 255

Activate your Sanctuary Membership 255

INDEX 257

Acknowledgements

My first thank you is reserved for Mantak Chia. It was his books on Taoist healing methods that provided the torch that, for me, lit the path forward in this work. Along the way, it was my good fortune to encounter wonderful teachers like Doctor Richard Tan, Kiiko Matsumoto, Stephen Birch, Daniel Atchison-Nevel, and Jeffrey Yuen. I thank them all for helping to expand my understanding of Chinese medicine. I'm grateful to my mentors in trance work, Doctor Rachel Hott and Steve Leeds, of the NLP Center of New York, for revealing to me the genius of Dr. Milton Erickson. In great part, it was his healing tales that provided me with a structure for how to proceed with this book.

A warm shout out goes to all wise women healers, past and present. Specifically, I thank my grandmother, Doña Regina, for showing me what a healer could be, and my mother, Maria, who exemplified the true meaning of strength. In regard to this book, I am grateful to Randy Rosenthal and Laura Shin for their insights in helping to bring it to fruition, and to Gina Ware of Here's the Cavalry for brilliantly collating the interactive experience that is the book and website. The wonderful graphics and cover design come courtesy of PRO100BBC and the photo is by Bethany Davis. You rock.

Finally, and most meaningfully, I'm beyond grateful to Carla Dawn, my amazing wife and partner in crime. Your love, encouragement, and faith in me carried me forward, even when I was unsure.

Preface

"I don't sleep."

Helene sits across from me at my desk, clutching an outsized pair of white sunglasses as if for dear life. She's 43 and the former editor of an art magazine.

"I'm glad you made it in," I reply. Her designer track suit hangs loosely on her, and she manages to send a gaunt smile my way. But there is fire in her eyes, and that is always a good sign.

"After my mini-breakdown," she continues, "I escaped LA and returned to New York to recoup. My doctors now have me on meds for high anxiety, IBS and depression. Tell the truth, am I broken?"

 "I've read your labs, and we can rule out that possibility. In fact, I know I can help you."

"You do acupuncture." Helene may as well have said, 'Great, you toss pebbles at the moon to try and change the tides." I mean, I want to believe, but…" her voice trails off.

"I appreciate the vote of faith," I reply, 'but that's not how acupuncture works. It might sound odd, but your symptoms are linked, like parts of a puzzle. Our training tells us that your body and mind are connected; as we treat one, the other invariably goes along for the ride as well."

Even as I say this, I sense one foot ascending a soapbox, and gingerly back down from it. "I think you'll find that, at the very least, acupuncture will reduce your symptoms greatly."

Seeming unimpressed by my assurances, Helene scans the worn, antique pharmacy sign from Japan gracing the wall beside a row of diplomas. If nothing else, her innate curiosity has been piqued.

"I'm told you do other therapies as well." Hedging her bets.

"Most acupuncturists also have training in herbology, or bodywork or nutrition. My focus is on sleep, so I might utilize neuroscience, trance work — whatever will help. There's a tool from neuroplasticity, which breaks up the fight-or-flight response that can inhibit healthy rest.",

"You are talking to Fight-or-Flight Central here." She leans in. "How does that work?"

"People who are prone to anxiety have good imaginations ..."

"I noticed, thank you very much." Helene releases the remnants of an ironic grin.

"Then maybe you've noticed how anxiety changes brain chemistry to create all sorts of odd associations."

"What kind of...odd associations?"

"Can you see how even momentary airplane turbulence might later show up as claustrophobia in elevators?"

"Enclosed spaces, feeling trapped. I could see how that's possible."

"What does it tell you, that sixty seconds in a balky airplane can create trauma?"

"It tells me we're susceptible to all kinds of horrible crap!" Helene lets out a small laugh.

"Yes, or maybe that the human mind is flexible. And just as we can short-circuit in one minute, with the right approach we can quickly bounce back, maybe better than before."

"Why don't we bounce back automatically?"

"Trauma gets trapped in the mind, and in muscle. Ideally, we want to release it in both places.

"How would someone do that?" Helene is now watching me intently.

"Getting a massage helps, as does acupuncture. You can also relax the nervous system on your own. One way is by using bilateral stimulation." I cross my arms and, splaying my hands across my upper chest, slowly tap a zone just below my collarbone with my index fingers. "Next time you feel a panic attack coming on," I tell her, "you could do this."

Helene becomes silent. She is either digesting what I said or else plotting a slyly executed escape.

On occasion, someone will ask me how I came to the work, and to this book. The roots of Rewired for Sleep are entwined with early memories in my grandmother's kitchen, in Argentina. I'd watch

Doña Regina peel an orange in a single, long curlicue before pinning the rind to a wall overnight to make digestive tea. I recall peeking from a doorway as she placed fire-heated glass cups on a person's back in order to treat asthma, or muscle pain. The mother of seven had an arsenal of wise-woman tools that had been handed down to her by her mother, all part of a great oral tradition that has largely fallen by the wayside.

When I was five, we immigrated to the USA, and natural medicine was soon forgotten. It wasn't until I was in my thirties and at the end of a career in music that my first love resurfaced, in the form of Chinese Medicine. When a rigorous four-year graduate program became available, I dove into it, graduating in 1995.

I was soon working in a clinic alongside MD's, physical therapists, and psychologists seeing multiple patients daily. While many of them recovered, a number of others plateaued. The practitioners with whom I worked were clearly talented, and yet, looking around me I saw many patients in clinic simply weren't getting better. My training soon clarified the problem: the focus was on symptom relief and prescription drugs rather than on lifestyle and stress reduction. After striking out on my own, I eventually came to specialize in treating insomnia. But as brilliant as Chinese medicine is, it hadn't been designed to repair insomnia arising from today's endless stressors and erratic treatment schedules. I saw that if I was truly going to help people sleep, I'd need to up my game so that they might help themselves.

This mini-revelation sparked a lengthy exploration into unconventional methods for treating sleep-related issues Most of them proved worthless. I collated the ones that remained with a single goal in mind: to provide for my patients—and the motivated reader—a roadmap to the innate "sleep doctor" that's inside us all. Rewired for Sleep was birthed over the next ten years.

Those seeking answers in the esoteric may be disappointed. The methods are reproducible and among those I use daily, in clinic; if one philosophy unites them, it is a universal idea that your body seeks balance. Every cell in your body wants that. When an internal problem disturbs sleep, your body is talking to you. It is saying, "We are off kilter and must do something different. Now." Your job is to listen, and then act on that information.

But maybe the inner voice is that of a skeptic, and right now it's saying, "hold on, we're not sold on this radical 'inner healer' pitch." And truly, why should you believe me? After all, modern medicine asks little of us except, perhaps, that we adhere to its latest commandment: Live better through chemistry. If my stomach is upset, I take a pill. If my back aches, I take another pill. If I can't sleep .... On the other side of the ledger, taking control of our own health may require effort, and insomnia sufferers are tired of jumping through hoops that, if past is prologue, rarely lead anyplace good.

Given the jumble of contradictory evidence around sleep, what I am proposing is that your inner skeptic has it only partly right. If the notion that you possess the tools necessary to sleep is a radical one, it's also as old as the human race.

"Come on," Helene says. "Let's do this."

Not long after Helene commits to twice-weekly treatments, she is sleeping through the night, waking once nightly to urinate. In time, her digestive issues and anxiety ease as well. The improvement in Helene's overall health is such that it surprises even her. Presently we'll see how Helene, and others who struggled with sleep, were able to take control of their lives.

It's possible that you too are sick and tired of being tired. Maybe you sense that, as the song says, "you've got the power," and you're ready to take it for a test drive. If so, then I invite you to accompany me on this trek to the Underworld, where sleep resides.

Introduction

As I began work on this book, my plan was to divide insomnia into its two broadest categories: difficulty getting to sleep, and difficulty staying asleep. It didn't take long to realize that it's rarely as black and white as those terms make it sound. As a result, the assorted tools I've provided were chosen for their ability to help almost anyone who may have problems sleeping.

The so-called "standard solution" invariably entails a prescription for drugs or open-ended talk therapy. They are poor substitutes for a long-lasting solution. It's no coincidence that many people tell me they feel abandoned by a medical system that appears to be deaf, dumb, and blind to their needs.

Here, in essence, is my reply: you have the skills to sleep. You just need to locate them. If you were going spelunking, you'd need strong rope, good boots, and a flashlight. Similarly, the inner trek to sleep requires patience, a cache of sturdy tools and a user's manual. The tools we'll use on our trek include:

• Chinese Medicine, including acupressure and internal strengthening exercises.

• Neuroplasticity, Neuro-Linguistic Programming and Cognitive Behavioral Therapy techniques

• Yogic breath work, guided visualization and easy-to-do forms of meditation (audio included).

- Sleep-positive food therapy, herbs, essential oils and supplements that replace chemicals.
- Body-Integrative methods: Meridian Tapping, Four-Step Trauma Relief, Reverse Spin and more.
- Progressive Muscle Relaxation and Autogenic Training to help calm the mind and relax the body.
- A commitment to self-care via affirmations, journaling and inner rewiring.

If the list seems wildly eclectic, know that it benefits you to have options. Certainly, if you had a broken bone and it needed setting, or if you were getting knee surgery, you'd want a codified system. But when it comes to finding sleep, a flexible, all-hands-on-deck approach is best. And since we currently have no universal switch that turns the mind on, or off, each of us requires customized tools.

Many of them you'll put into use immediately; others may require practice. As someone who spent years practicing a musical instrument for four hours a day, the "p" word still makes me itch. Still, I urge you to view your body as your instrument. If you've played sports, crocheted, cooked — anything requiring a bit of skill — then you know that repetition is core to getting it right. Give your precious instrument its due; it will lead you to sleep.

How Long Before I'm Fixed?

It depends. If sleeplessness is due to a recent change of home, or a job, or perhaps a relationship breakup, the chances are your sleep rhythm will return relatively quickly. More often, the problem has gained traction slowly over years. For now, let's call Time an ally. If after shifting your routine for, say a month, your sleep had improved, would you call that time well spent? In a world where time is money, I call that a good return on your investment. Priorities matter.

A Word About Method, and a Caveat

The use of patients' stories to instruct is not new. We may look back to Chunyu Yin in 100 BC to see where physicians first used case histories. But it was in the Ming dynasty that texts consisting mainly of case histories detailing multiple modalities began to appear. As described by the physician, Wang Ji, a diversity of styles in almost every aspect of medicine allowed a patient to dictate what sort of medicine he or she would take part in.

This bit of history has relevance for us today. We can continue to lean solely on Western medicine and wait for it to fix us. We can also explore systems of healing that have stood the test of time: yoga, acupuncture, qi gong, bodywork, trance, and nutrition among them. Implicit in the concept of choice is a profound, and simple, idea, "take what you need and leave the rest". It is there, at the crossroads where caveat meets offer, that increased vitality wins the day.

More Caveats

Some sleep disorders require professional treatment. If you struggle with Circadian Rhythm Sleep Disorder, Sleep Paralysis, Narcolepsy, or Somnambulism, these tools may fall short for your needs. If you find that to be the case, I urge you to seek out professional help for these problems, or for any that may require a diagnosis leading to the use of Chinese herbs (more on them, later.)

The other caveat is this: the case histories tend to reflect success stories. You probably won't be shocked if I tell you that not every patient returns to normal sleeping habits. Some are disheartened after only unspectacular change; others don't connect with the methods offered. If I do not display those as well, it's because I saw little to be gleaned from their inclusion.

Regain Control of Your Sleep

It's my hope that as you do the exercises, you'll regain your innate ability to enter that other good night. You see, healthy sleep is that important. If interrupted sleep corrodes our vitality, then a night's rest restores us. If unwanted side-effects are the body's push back against chemical band-aids, the message is that your body deserves better. Along the way old aches ease, and a once-sluggish metabolism burns off weight while we sleep. It's true that self-empowerment is a traveled phrase. Still, I urge you to grab hold of its underlying sentiment as if it were a compass, and let sleep be your True North. Hold on to that inner compass: It'll get you where you want to go.

How to use this book:

As you read Rewired for Sleep, you needn't try to absorb the tools for self-repair all at once, or even decide which ones might best suit you. My goal in using case histories was to provide you with a loose sense of how these tools have worked for others, and how they may do the same for you. Let them percolate. Then, when you're ready, explore and experiment with the 28-Day Insomnia Repair Program to create your own unique program of sleep repair.

You can follow the program using the book or head over to the website at rewiredforsleep.com and explore The Rewired Sanctuary. This online supplement to the book offers many resources including a daily interactive version of the 28-Day

Program, simple tutorials and sleep journal prompts. Perhaps most important, you'll have access to powerful audio recordings for meditations, exercises and guided visualizations. My goal in designing Rewired Sanctuary was to help make your trek back to sleep as easy as possible. I hope you'll use it to your benefit.

The good news is that when you purchased your copy of Rewired for Sleep, you gained a complimentary membership of The Rewired Sanctuary. All you need to do is activate it. The instructions and activation code can be found at the end of the book.

PART I:

Sleeping in the Material World

"Dig a well before you are thirsty."

– Chinese proverb

Chapter 1:

Insomniac's Guide to the Underworld

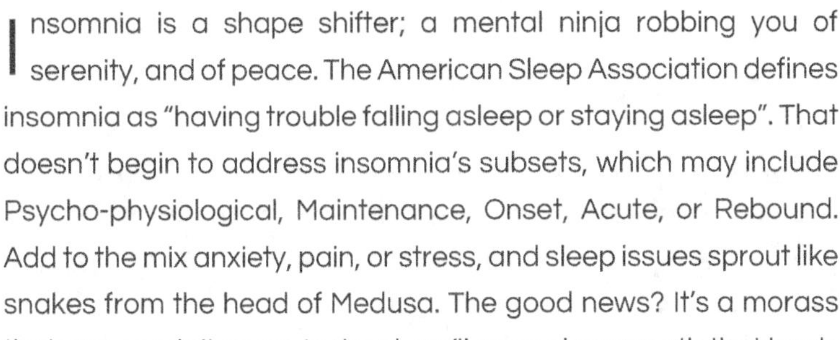

Insomnia is a shape shifter; a mental ninja robbing you of serenity, and of peace. The American Sleep Association defines insomnia as "having trouble falling asleep or staying asleep". That doesn't begin to address insomnia's subsets, which may include Psycho-physiological, Maintenance, Onset, Acute, or Rebound. Add to the mix anxiety, pain, or stress, and sleep issues sprout like snakes from the head of Medusa. The good news? It's a morass that you needn't cross. Instead, we'll soon clear a path that leads to the door of the underworld, where sleep resides.

A Map of the Map

The first steps will be to identify your main sensor, and then set up a sleep journal. Next, you'll start removing barriers to healthy rest using breath work and Meridian Tapping. We'll discuss sleep-positive food, supplements and herbs, after which you'll access tools to reduce anxiety such as Reverse Spin and Six Healing Sounds. Throughout, you'll learn techniques that combat the squirmy, sleepless mind. Much of the information is supported by recordings you can listen to on your trek to sleep.

If it all sounds overwhelming, know that almost every journey feels that way at first. But each journey also begins with a first step, so: breathe in, and take that first step into the V-A-K Sensor. As you'll soon see, your response to this exercise will come in handy once you start using the various modules.

Exercise 1: The V-A-K Sensor

You can listen to The V-A-K Sensor at rewiredforsleep.com/the-deeper-levels.

We all have a main sensory filter through which we perceive the world. For our purposes, we tend to perceive things Visually, Auditorily (through sound) or Kinesthetically via feeling (thus V-A-K). A person who is predominantly Visual ("I see what you're saying," "I get the picture") responds best to pictures, diagrams, and charts. An Auditory type ("I hear you"; "that rings a bell") is sparked by sound, or voice. A person who's mainly Kinesthetic will say, "I like a hands-on approach"; "that feels right." They are huggers.

If you suspect that you are a combination of all three, you're right. And yet, you also use one sensor more than you do the others. The exercise will show you the one you naturally lean into. As I indicated, knowing your main sensor will help you later to better utilize the various tools we are going to access.

Record the exercise, have someone read it to you, or listen to it at rewiredforsleep.com/the-deeper-levels.

The three words to remember are: Calm, Candle, and Breath.

1. Close your eyes. Say the word "calm" out loud.

2. Now, say "calm" softly, under your breath.

3. With your eyes closed, softly repeat "calm" in your mind, for about ten seconds: "Calm, calm, calm," almost like a faint,

distant bell you're hearing.

4. On a scale of one to ten, with ten being extremely relaxed and one being barely relaxed at all, rate how it felt to you:

   ____

5. With your eyes closed, imagine a candle flickering. With eyes still shut, imagine that candle flickering for a good fifteen seconds.

6. Now, on a scale of one to ten, with ten being relaxed and one being barely relaxed at all, rate that mini-exercise:

   ____

7. Take a gentle, full breath in, hold it for two seconds, and exhale.

8. With your eyes closed, notice the sound of your breath going in, and going out.

9. Notice the sound and feeling of your breath for about twenty seconds.

10. On a scale of one to ten, with ten being relaxed and one being tense, rate the mini-exercise _________

Note: If you chose Sensor 1, you're primarily an Auditory type. If you picked number 2, you tend to be Visual. If you identified with number 3, you tend to perceive the world kinesthetically. Which sensor did you find the most calming?

How did it feel to relax your nervous system using your own mind?

The Power of Touch

The use of pressure on the body in order to affect a therapeutic change is as old as mankind. The systemization of that therapy is part of Chinese Medicine, an oceanic system of health into which we'll soon dip a toe. As we continue on our trek to the Underworld, we'll gather numerous acupoints that help ignite healthy sleep. Place each one in your bag of tools for such time as you might have need for it.

The Power of Words

We know that words carry emotional weight. An offhand rebuke at the wrong moment, from the right person, can twist us up inside even when we know better. But what about the words we use with ourselves? Words like insomnia, anxiety, and pain hold little weight. Attach the possessive noun "my," and psyche says, "It's mine. I own this." It's natural to want to keep a possession, even when it doesn't serve us. But as we become mindful of the words we use, the subconscious mind gets the message. This beneficial attitude becomes ingrained, and unwanted states fall away.

 A statement such as, "I'm an insomniac," leaves little room for other options. But if we say, "I'm experiencing anxiety" or, "I'm going through sleep issues," this implies a capacity for change. Brain Central picks up on this idea that we're just passing through some bad lands on our way to sleep, and runs with the idea that it, indeed, has options.

We can also make inroads by shifting time frame. "I am anxious," or even, "I have anxiety" are statements that leave little room for change to occur. When we say, "I've experienced anxiety" (even if it is ongoing), we relegate it to the past while leaving open the door for solutions — something the anxious mind tries to avoid at all costs. By using words that nudge us away from an anxious state, to a more manageable one of worry, we align ourselves with a state that is already hardwired into our DNA. We tend to go from problem to solution, and then back to problem again with barely time in between. We worry a problem until we solve it. It's what we do.

Exercise 2: My Friend John/Jane

Anxiety hides in corners, telling us that something — we're never sure what--is not as it should be. By shining a light on those dark places in our mind, we can separate the formlessness of anxiety from a real problem. By defining a problem and then tracking its trajectory, we detach from anxiety in a healthy way. It's a four-step process, that goes from defining the problem to generating solutions.

In step 1 we define the problem (i.e., I just can't sleep at night; my brain won't turn off...)

In step two we utilize detachment in order to generate solutions that we might otherwise not have.

In a sentence, what would you tell a friend who asked you for a solution to this problem?

Solution A (Ex: Exercise so that at night you're exhausted and will fall asleep)

Solution B (Ex:Try CBD oil or herbs. Use Remake Your Day, or Move the Voice)

Solution C (Ex: Learn how to relax your muscles with Progressive Muscle Relaxation)

Which of these solutions seems like the best one?

____

On a scale of 1 to 10 (ten being most doable), how doable is this solution?

____

When you are feeling stuck, My Friend John/Jane, can help you get unstuck.

Sleep Journal

If you were about to trek into unfamiliar terrain, you'd hire a guide. For our discussion, a sleep journal can get you back on track if you stray from it. Set up a sleep journal on your computer, or in a physical three-ring binder with tabs on the side, whichever works best. One section, Strategies, will contain the exercises with which you most resonate. Mark a section "Journaling." That's where you'll record your progress. If you've got little to input now, that will change.

Sleep Journaling:

1) Exercise(s) I did today

2) Today's Goals

3) What I did differently

4). Awareness for Today

5). Acceptance for Today

6). Actions for Today

7). Actualization: Hours Slept

At first, question # 7 may feel like an emotional landmine. That number will begin to rise, and probably sooner than later.

Chapter 2:

Under Pressure: The Cop and the Restless Leg

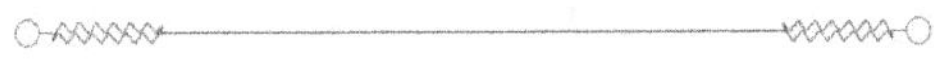

Eamon, 36, sports an oversized Rangers jersey and big, generous laugh. A New York City policeman, his chief complaint is Restless Leg Syndrome (RLS). This fairly common malady wakes him nightly and keeps him awake, often for hours at a clip. Characterized by a need to move one's body to stop uncomfortable sensations, it usually affects the legs. With a bit of prodding, Eamon reveals that he is also anxious and suffers with acid reflux.

As we chat, I check his radial pulse. It's bouncing around under my fingertips like a tightrope wire, verifying that Eamon's nervous system is overloaded. I then examine the surface of his tongue to get a better picture of what's happening on an internal level. A furry, yellow coating in the center of it is indicative of heat in his digestive tract, even as the reddish tip further underlines emotional displacement. Together, they provide me with clues as to how I'll begin treatment.

"There's nothing really wrong with me," he proclaims: "It's just all these thoughts swirling through me at night, you know?"

This is his first encounter of the acupuncture kind, and he's taking in every detail of the treatment room. Given the work he does, I imagine he is generally watchful. He comments how unlike a standard doctor's visit this is, even as I begin placing tiny pins along his arms and legs.

"The pins," he says, "what do they do?"

"They release chemicals that relax the muscles and help your mind unwind." That absurdly incomplete explanation will have to suffice for now. I'm in a zone that demands focus.

"Didn't even feel that one going in," he says, starting a running commentary. "That one I felt, but not bad. What's THAT one do?" And so it goes. When I'm done, I leave him on the table to let the therapy take effect.

Thirty minutes later I re-enter the room. Eamon is asleep, a common occurrence during treatment. After waking him I remove the pins, place them in a sharps container — pins are used once and then discarded--and retreat so he may gather himself. By the time I return, he's fully dressed and studying a wall chart of the myriad acupoints on the human ear.

He turns to face me, a mildly loopy grin on his face.

"I feel pretty good." He sounds surprised. "Anything I can do to, you know, help myself?"

"There's an acupressure point you can massage to help you get back to sleep."

Acupressure for Sleep

The first point we'll gather for our trek is Anmian, which means peaceful sleep in Chinese. Often used in the treatment of insomnia, it's also helpful in easing agitation and anxiety.

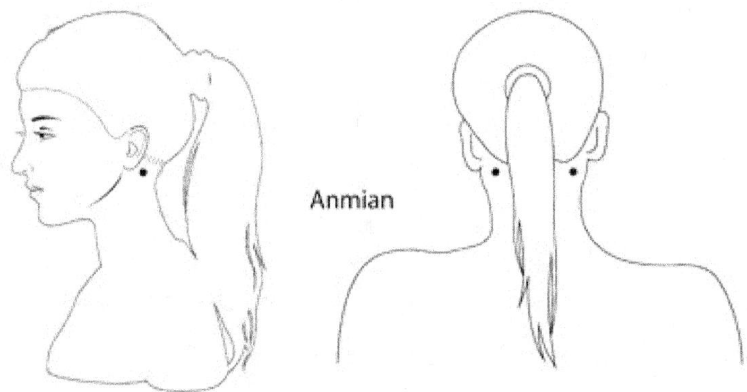

Find Anmian behind the ear near the earlobe, by a small rounded bone which points downwards (mastoid process). Place your finger on the protruding part of the bone and slide it backward, until you find a slight depression. From there, slide the finger diagonally up and back towards the base of your skull. Place a finger or thumb on both sides and rotate it twenty-four times in each direction. Whether it feels relaxing or achy, lightly massaging it will benefit you.

"Breathe into it."

Furrowing his brow, he digs his thumbs in the area. "Right there! I'll try this tonight."

During his fourth session he tells me the leg spasms have eased, but anxiety is still a clamp in his chest. I prescribe a liver detox decoction and hand him a printout for The Five, Five, and Five exercise.

"And I should do what with this?" he asks.

"They're exercises that gets those negative thoughts in your head out into the light."

"Good luck with that," he murmurs.

Exercise 3: The Five, Five, and Five

1. Take three deep breaths. On the first breath, let your shoulders slump down. On the second breath, clench and then unclench your jaw. On the third breath, close your eyes for five minutes. As you breathe rhythmically, imagine a calming image, such as an awesome sunrise, or a tree with roots that nourish you. Or, you can create your own image (V, K).

2. For five minutes, focus on a positive word, such as "Easy," or "Comfort." Don't worry if your mind wanders, that's natural. Return to the word you've chosen (A).

3. For five minutes, jot down whatever comes to mind without judgment, letting your hand go. If an image, feeling, or thought you're not "proud of" comes up, keep writing (A, K).

I give him magnesium, a natural mineral that is commonly used for RLS. It's known to have a dual effect of relaxing muscles due to cramping, and to help people sleep as well. In one 2012 study involving 46 seniors with insomnia, those who took 500-mg magnesium supplements for eight weeks appeared to improve some insomnia symptoms, including sleep efficiency, sleep time, ability to fall asleep as well as early morning awakening.

Natural sources of magnesium include pumpkin seeds, sunflower seeds and sesame seeds, along with leafy greens such as spinach and Swiss chard. Many people find that taking a bath with Epsom salts before bed helps them fall asleep.

Over four weeks' time, and after multiple treatments, Eamon says the RLS is now infrequent and milder in intensity, allowing him to sleep through the night. As for the anxiety, he says the work we've been doing has been helpful. The acid reflux has also eased, but Eamon declines further treatment, opting to rely on his gastroenterologist instead.

With Eamon's blessing, I tape tiny stimuli to his ear, as shown on the diagram. Their intended effect is to enhance his digestive system, and I advise him to gently massage the points after meals. We'll delve into these tools for self-help, among many others, soon enough.

Digestive Issues

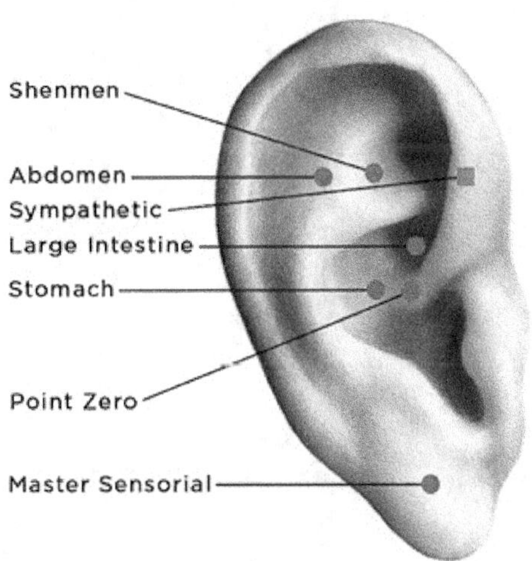

Chapter 3:

The Barriers to Sleep, & Sleep Hygiene

The Barriers to Sleep

The galaxy of sleep issues that we refer to as "insomnia" seems to be one that is expanding. Sleeplessness affects four out of ten people, and half of them chronically. It might appear for any number of reasons, but there are certain barriers to sleep that I've identified, and which I'll return to time and again. They are anxiety, digestive issues, stress, chemical problems, and pain*.

We might struggle with several barriers at once, creating "bleed through." You're worried about your job, are anxious and can't sleep. Stress leads to stomach issues and difficulty resting. Indigestion flairs up, and the night is lost. This also works in reverse: break down one barrier and others often fall, domino-like. Lower your stress, and stomach tension often eases as well. In that case, sleep is rarely far away. Much of what we'll do is intended to break down the barriers.

*Pain is a significant barrier to healthy sleep. While we can reduce its impact using the methods found here, it's not the focus of this book. I suggest you seek out a professional for help with it. Acupuncture is an effective treatment solution, when performed by a licensed practitioner.

That having been said, Large Intestine 4 (LI4) is a powerful point that can help to reduce discomfort. Gentle massage helps diminish headaches, cold symptoms, constipation and problems on the face (toothache, allergies, eye problems, rhinitis, hay fever, acne). LI4 is located on the highest spot of the muscle when the thumb and index fingers are brought close together. Move your thumb along the bone, find the most painful spot. and massage it. Not to be used if pregnant.

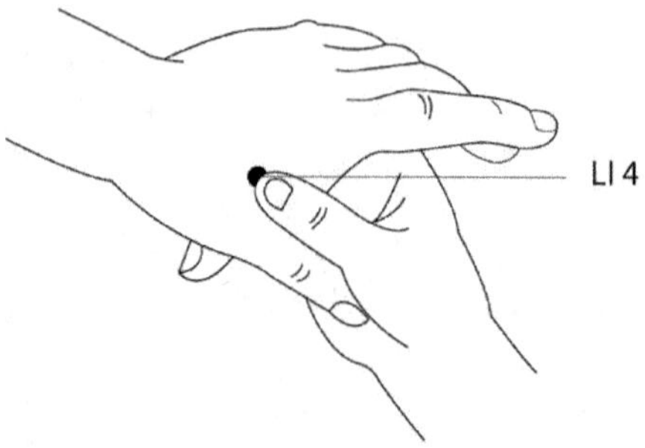

Sleep Hygiene

- Part of Cognitive Behavioral Therapy (CBT), sleep hygiene refers to a loose set of sleep rules that is often recommended by doctors as a template for relieving insomnia. If you're already familiar with the list, go through it anyway; repetition is always helpful.

- Stick to the twenty-minute rule: If you've been lying in bed awake for twenty minutes, get up and do something else. Some people tidy up the room or the house. You might write in your sleep journal. Keep the lights at a low level, even if you're reading. And forget your phone!

- Try not to lay there tossing and turning, as it can make for an antagonistic relationship with your bed. If hanging out on your sofa is an option, do so, then return to the bed when you feel you can sleep.

- Don't read or watch TV in bed: Doing either one can make insomnia worse. People without sleep problems can do those things, but your bed should be for two things only: sleep and sex.

- Napping: Experts are split on this. Cognitive Behavioral Therapists tend to say that naps inhibit night time sleep and should be avoided. Some people find that a solid 20-30-minute snooze can improve mood, alertness, and performance.

- Remove ALL artificial light including the light on your alarm clock, TV light, phone, etc. If that's impossible then duct tape over lights. Blackout curtains or an eye mask are helpful to guard against outside artificial light. The most restorative levels of sleep coincide with the highest levels of melatonin and the lowest point of core body temperature. Exposure to bright (artificial) light sources — in particular, television or computer screens — shortly before going to bed, results in a delayed increase in melatonin. This, in turn, causes difficulties with falling asleep or superficial sleep and can lead to waking in the middle of the night.

- Exercise: We know that exercise benefits sleep. What matters for us is when. There is a twenty-four-hour cycle, known as Circadian Rhythm, for various physiological, behavioral, and biochemical processes that occur within the body. Body temperature typically has two peaks and two troughs per 24-hour cycle. You're most likely to fall asleep when your body temperature is dropping, or on the downward cycle — mid-afternoon and at night. Exercise increases body temperature, and when you do it too late in the day your body temperature will take longer to drop. Therefore, the optimal time to exercise is four to five hours before bedtime, or in the morning.

- Temperature: Studies show the optimal temperature for sleep is between 65-68 degrees.

- Sound: White noise, the sound of rain, or the ocean may help, so long as it lulls you to sleep and doesn't energize you. Make your wake-up alarm tone a gentle sound.

- Set a Time: This is a tough one, given that we all have different schedules and lifestyles. Ideally, be in bed by 10 p.m. to enhance your body's recuperation time. If you're not home before 9 p.m. and need time to unwind or hang out with your family, set a time and stick with it.

- Bath: Before bed, take a hot bath in Epsom salts and eucalyptus oil (Jones' 23 oil is terrific), especially if you have any sort of muscle ache.

- Make a List: Before going to bed, make a list of up to eight things that you want to get done the next day. Don't get too specific or think about it too much, and don't get hung up on any one item. In fact, you probably won't even get half that list completed. Write the list and then mentally let it go. Use these words: These are tomorrow's concerns, not tonight's.

Daniel's Extended Sleep Hygiene List

- Nature: Spend time outside daily for at least thirty minutes. Ideally, you're walking barefoot on dirt, grass, or rocks. This seemingly minor activity is very important for the body, mind, and spirit.

- Sex: You could do worse than masturbating or engaging in some full-on sex to relieve anxiety or stress. It is natural, and it's your body, so have at it. (Note: As several women throughout history have noted, men often fall off the face of the earth after sex; in this divine comedy, women are often energized by it. Adjust as needed.)

- Polarity: Use the earth's magnetic polarity. Simply position the bed so your head points north and your feet toward the south.

The following exercises are available to Rewired Sanctuary members as printable Sleep Journal worksheets on my website as the starting point for the 28-Day Insomnia Repair Program. https://rewiredforsleep.com/barriers-to-sleep

Which of these barriers do you feel might be more difficult to change?

Which barriers do you think will be the easiest to change?

Which one do you want to start with?

Does tonight feel like a good time to start?

If not tonight, then when?

The Big Lie About Sleep: You Need Eight Hours

Throughout history, people have awakened for an hour or two in the night. For many of us, breaking up the night's sleep is the biologically "normal" thing to do. In pre-industrial times, a strict eight-hours sleep was not the norm. The industrial revolution changed all that. Suddenly, people needed to be in bed at a particular time so they could get up and go to work at a prescribed hour.

What's worse, "Early to bed, early to rise" can be harmful to the psyche. If we believe we're supposed to get eight "solid" hours of sleep, anything less and we might feel cheated. "This is wrong!" we tell ourselves. "I shouldn't be awake!" Stress hormones hit the body like a shot of espresso, and sleep suffers as a result. But if we know it's normal to wake up for a while at night, we're actually giving our modern brain a way back to sleep. Maybe sleeping straight through the night isn't "normal" for you.

Removing More Barriers to Sleep

Question: Are you ready to get rid of the source of your insomnia?

___________________.

The answer may be obvious, even a no-brainer. But the question could spark a story lurking in a corner of your mind as to why you can't sleep. If such a story emerges, release it; it wasn't yours. The following questions are meant to clarify the level of your willingness to win at the sleep game.

Am I willing, at this moment, for my sleep to be different, and better, than it is right now?

Yes ___________ No ___________

Am I ready to let go of unease and stress in my life?

Yes___________ No ___________

Deep down, do I feel I'd be sacrificing something by letting go of stress?

Yes___________ No___________

If the answer is yes, what would I be sacrificing?

Is that sacrifice more important to me than my health?

Yes ___________ No ___________

Do I owe it to myself to do *whatever* it takes to start sleeping better short of taking a pill?

Yes _________ No _________

For today, am I willing to be willing to make healthy sleep a priority?

Yes _________ No _________

Can I allow myself to imagine that I could sleep better than I am now?

In 3 months? _________ In 1 month? _________

Next, we'll examine the Evil Twins of sleep deprivation: stress and unbalanced lifestyle.

Chapter 4

Stress and Lifestyle

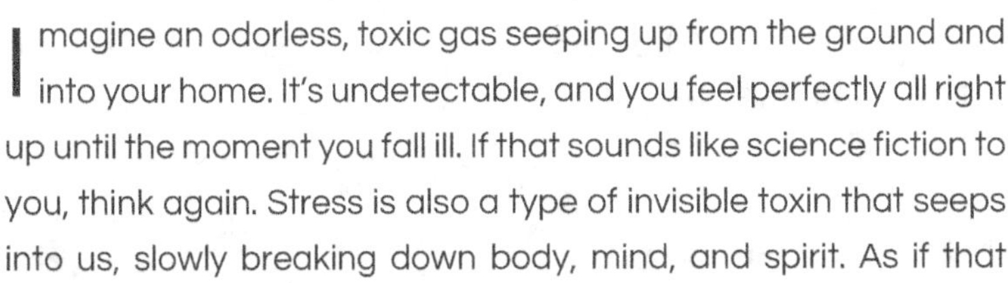

Imagine an odorless, toxic gas seeping up from the ground and into your home. It's undetectable, and you feel perfectly all right up until the moment you fall ill. If that sounds like science fiction to you, think again. Stress is also a type of invisible toxin that seeps into us, slowly breaking down body, mind, and spirit. As if that weren't bad enough, stress is also a real sleep killer. It's time we began chipping away at it.

David and the Spaghetti-Tangled Mind

David, 46, sits across from me, nattily attired in a seersucker suit and blue polka-dot bowtie. Bushy eyebrows pop up from behind tortoise-rim glasses when he is animated, which is often. A lawyer, he is now "making bank" on Wall Street. Long, stressful workdays often segue into late meals and subsequent acid reflux. The twenty pounds he's been trying to lose for two years have edged north of forty. It's no coincidence that David, a poor sleeper, was recently diagnosed as having sleep apnea.

> "I'm up for making lifestyle changes," says David. "I just can't do crazy sacrifices right now. Here's how I see it. My mind's a computer with a virus that's programmed to fail at sleep, and I'm powerless to change the program. I get in bed at night and think to myself, tonight I'm going to sleep, damn it! And … nothing."

In a way, David has the right idea. There are chemical messengers in the brain, known as neurotransmitters, that carry signals to receptor sites affecting heart rate, mood, appetite, sleep, and fear. The neurotransmitters that carry stress-producing chemicals attach to receptor sites that support them. They bind together like branches of a tree; as those branches grow together, they get stronger, and more entrenched.

The result? The word "sleep" releases stress hormone (I can't sleep!). Neurotransmitter finds receptor (can't sleep, AGAIN), the virus programming gets lit up (I'm a failure AND I can't sleep), and David is off to the insomnia races all in about half-a-second.

"That's very interesting," David says. "Question is, how do I start sleeping again?"

"We use positive experiences to enlist 'feel good' chemicals, such as endorphin, and pave over the negative ones. This way, we build new neural pathways that support sleep." David raises an eyebrow in response. I can't blame him for his skeptical attitude.

Indeed, if repairing our spaghetti-tangled brain sounds like a tall order, we're capable of that, and more. We're a survivor species. For proof, we need look no further than to our nervous system, its two halves chugging away in see-saw fashion. The sympathetic nervous system (SNS), revs us up, and the parasympathetic (PNS) calms us down. Normally the SNS and PNS toggle back and forth depending on life events. It's always been thus.

In prehistoric times, the SNS provided the energy we needed to attack a woolly mammoth and the jolt necessary to run, in case the plan fizzled. But if we triumphed, we would drag our prize to our lair, eat … and sleep. By then the PNS would have released the chemical norepinephrine to slow heartbeat and respiration, and to promote healing. Our nervous system was built to absorb the day's stressors, relax, sleep, and then do it all again the next day.

In our post-industrial, post-modern world, damage comes from a procession of small stressors. They are inconstant and arrive as time pressure, blinking clocks, endless emails, and ever-newer technology. We absorb one, but then ten more replace it. This constant onslaught impacts on every part of our being. And it really messes with our sleep

The Anti-Anxiety Anchor (K)

It's usually when we're most stressed out that we forget the important things. Like breathing. Having a physical "anchor" can help remind us to regain a sense of calm. This reminder to break a negative state can be as simple as snapping your fingers. When you are feeling the first hints of anxiety, snap your fingers twice. That will be your reminder to take a deep breath, followed by two more breaths. This is an example of making a connection to your body in order to push back against anxiety. Repetition helps. I invite you to do this simple encoding process five times a day for a week. Anxious? Snap your fingers twice and breathe.

Lifestyle

For our purposes, the word "lifestyle" encompasses our relationship with food, work, others, sex, exercise, and ourselves. Everything we do releases chemicals that create pools of electrical energy. When we're too festive or work too hard, eat nutrition-free food or sit too much, that energy stagnates, creating internal problems that can really gum up the works. But since we are a survivor species, our body is built to tolerate these mini-abuses for a long time.

Suddenly, the psyche exclaims, "Enough!" It expresses discontent with the way we're treating it by pinging out anxiety, an achy neck or back, or loss of sleep. There may be an urge to abuse daiquiris or donuts, or to throw our hands in the air and say, "It's just aging!" We ignore those annoying blips, but then recall an ad touting a pill that makes all the bad stuff go away. And down the rabbit-hole we go.

"I know lifestyle's a factor," says David. "It's what Charlotte's always telling me. Truth? I need carbs to function at a high level for work. Without my carbs, I'm sunk."

There are times when an acupuncturist has to keep mouth shut, head down, and just do the work. The treatment I use with David is meant to lower stress and help control his appetite. In the end, though, I need to enlist David. Whether I'll get his help is another matter.

Schedule a Worry Session

Pick a designated time of day to address your problems. If a negative thought enters your mind outside of your scheduled worry session, jot it down so you can more calmly address it during your scheduled worry time. Then return to your day. NOTE: schedule your worry session before 7 p.m. for best results.

Breathe! (Abdominal Breathing)

I try and observe how patients breathe. If they're breathing incorrectly, I show them the right way. This instruction is doubly important for those who lean toward anxiety, as their breathing tends to be shallow. Given the ragged quality of David's respiration, I offer to help him correct it.

"I know how to breathe," he says. "I've been breathing my whole life. And what's it got do with getting a night's sleep?"

"Just everything. Shallow breathing decreases oxygen intake; it distorts mood, makes us fuzzy headed. Most of us inhale by puffing out our chest and tucking in the gut. Breathe as you naturally do, and notice what your shoulders are doing."

As David inhales, his shoulders rise six inches; he looks at me quizzically.

"The air stays high in your chest," I say. "It's how most of us breathe, especially when we're under stress. It's how we breathe when danger is nearby. It's survival mode breathing."

I have him lay face-up on the treatment table, palms flat on his belly.

"Now breathe down past your lungs, so your hands rise and fall as you breathe. Inhale into your belly for a count of four. Hold it for a count of two and then breathe out for four. People who do sports or yoga breathe this way, as do actors. It's called abdominal breathing, or belly breathing."

"I feel weird," David says. "Lightheaded."

"That's natural at first. Soon, the twenty-three thousand breaths you take daily will give you more energy; it's how we breathed when we were babies."

"You think we might have been shown this in kindergarten?" he says. I nod my head in agreement.

"At bedtime," he adds, "my mind swirls with the day's wins, losses, and betrayals. It's like there's this voice that ambushes me just as I'm slipping under the covers." If you're in bed at night and hear a voice rattling about in your head — whether it's that of a parent or a boss, or even your own — know that its mission is to damage your rest. Your mission is to displace that voice, and this exercise does that.

Exercise 4: Move the Voice (V-A)

"Close your eyes," I say, "and take three belly breaths. Now, locate the negative voice in your head. The judgmental voice. Can you hear, or feel it?"

"It's Pops," he says matter-of-factly.

"Is it any place in particular: upper right side? Lower right?"

"Upper left side of my head."

"Good. Now open your eyes, take a deep breath in."

He does as I ask.

"Now, call up the voice of someone you trust." He nods in assent. "Whose voice is it?"

"Charlotte. My wife. My amazing wife."

"Close your eyes again. Notice where that voice is located in your head."

"Ahh. She's in the lower right quadrant of my head, whispering to me."

"Great. Now move Pop's voice, from the left upper quadrant to the lower right side where Charlotte's voice sat. Let me know when you've done that."

I wait. He nods his head.

"Notice how that voice sounds now. Is it the same, or has it changed?"

"It's softer. It's no longer grinding and harsh. How weird is that."

"Not so weird. You unplugged the negative voice from your head."

"Charlotte," David says at his treatment four days later, "claims she sees a difference." Like he has no skin in the game. "But late at night, when I"m alone, in my thoughts, it's still hard for me to let go. Whether it's a comment someone made, or something I should have done, my mind can chew that bone until it's dust. Know what I mean?"

"Yes, I do. The good thing? You can 'Remake Your Day.'"

Exercise 5: Remake Your Day

As you're turning in for the night, take a minute to go over your day. This is one time when you can focus on those things that went wrong in the previous twenty-four hours. It's the first step toward remaking them in your mind to the way you'd want them to be. By overlaying a positive image over a negative one, you rewire your brain's neural transmitters to create a more positive result in the future. How is that possible?

Neuroscience makes clear that your brain is made up of billions of interconnected cells called neurons, which hold all your memories, produce your feelings, and initiate all of your actions. Neurons are flexible, and capable of change. Just as the cells on your arm can regenerate to heal a wound, you can replace neurons that lead to unproductive belief systems ("I can't sleep," "I'm anxious") with others that are more beneficial ("I am able to sleep," "I am calm," "I control my mind"). If you are thinking to yourself, "that's great, but how can this help me sleep?", we'll put this information to use in Chapter Seven.

"Sounds like an exercise in wishful thinking," David says. "Got no time for that in my business."

"You play golf?

"Now that, I've got time for." His grin displays a healthy gap between his upper front teeth. "I'm actually pretty good, too."

"This is the same technique golf coaches use to help people work on their swing. Music teachers have their students practice an arpeggio in their mind. By the time they're at a piano, muscle memory has created a new neural pathway. - When you're doing Remake Your Day, enlist all of your V-A-K sensors for support."

"What if an image comes up that I don't want"

"If that happens, recall, or imagine, one you'd prefer and work backward. Use V-A-K with actions, positive words, and feelings. Soon, a positive scenario will begin to embed itself in muscle memory."

"Then what?" says David.

"Then rinse, repeat, and rest. There's an acupoint that helps to relax you at night."

"Great! Charlotte eats this stuff up."

"I'm sure it's Charlotte who could profit from it."

"I see what you did there."

"The point is called Yintang, or Seal Hall. It helps ease insomnia and anxiety. It relaxes the nervous system, eases headaches, sinusitis, vertigo, and dizziness. It's between the eyebrows, in the bend where the bridge of the nose meets the forehead.

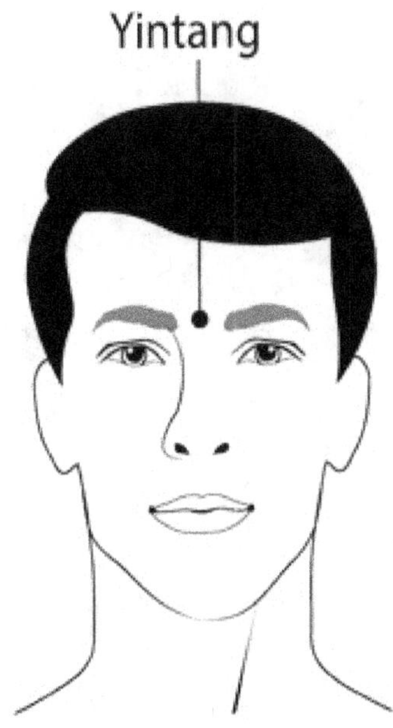

"Place the tip of an index finger on it and gently rotate your finger twenty-four times. As you practice belly breathing, imagine you're exhaling through Yintang."

"Really?" David plays to his self-admitted caricature by rolling his eyes. But he reports that breathing through Yintang has the effect of centering him — even as the idea of it is ludicrous. But that's the thing: it doesn't matter if we find the ideas ludicrous. They work.

I prescribe magnolia bark (Hou Po). The herb boosts levels of GABA, a neurotransmitter that increases the amount of time you spend in REM sleep while reducing the time it takes to fall asleep. It's also an adrenaline inhibitor, meaning it suppresses high levels of cortisol and thereby reduces stress/anxiety. As if that were not enough, magnolia bark eases abdominal bloating, pain and nausea, and regulates the appetite. [**Note**: It is contraindicated for pregnancy or those planning surgery.]

David also starts taking Siberian Ginseng. Often called an "adaptogen," the term is used to describe substances that can strengthen the body and increase resistance to daily stress. **Note:** not all ginseng is the same. Korean ginseng, for instance, is considered a "hot" herb and will keep you awake at night. As always, when it comes to Asian herbs, you are best served seeing a qualified herbalist.

Break-in: Under 3rd Toe

This control point for blood pressure comes from a Japanese tradition. It is indicated for anxiety, palpitations, insomnia, temperature imbalances, and sweating. You may massage it or apply heat (instructions for that are in a later chapter).

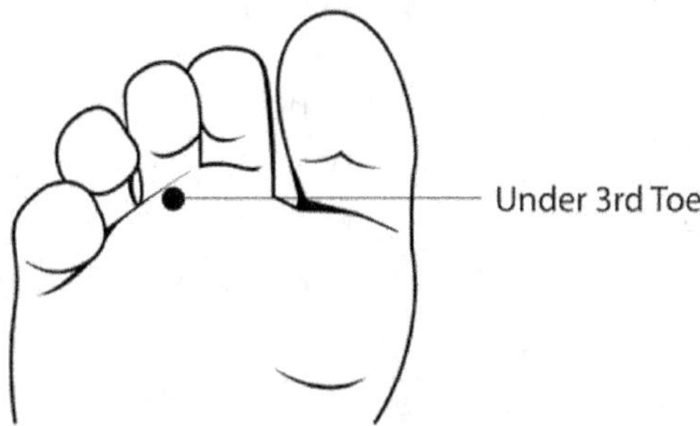

David does breath work, utilizes the anti-anxiety anchor, and massages Yintang and Under 3rd Toe. At night, he does Remake Your Day. He continues to receive acupuncture treatments, as well.

The upshot is that he is falling asleep soon after his head touches the pillow. Equally important, he's waking energized the next morning. David renews his gym membership. As often happens when people take their exercise regimens seriously, he can't help but see the damage that carbs do.

David walks in to my office with a determined look in his eyes I've not seen before.

"Let's talk food."

We focus on sleep-positive food (see Chapter Ten), even as I guide him to a holistic nutritionist. Over the next four months, David sheds twenty-six pounds thanks in part to going to the gym, but mainly due to making informed food choices. That he's sleeping more deeply makes a difference as well.

"I'm building muscle mass," he tells me, "faster than I did when I was twenty." He flexes a bicep as proof.

One of the most important naturally occurring anabolic hormones (those that promote muscle growth) is Growth Hormone (GH). As it turns out, the release of GH is tightly linked with sleep. Although we haven't yet discussed the stages of sleep, know that 70% of GH is secreted during Stage 3 sleep, and that the total amount of GH released in your body is directly correlated with how much Stage 3 sleep you get, or don't get. Your ability to release weight in a meaningful manner is very much dependent on your ability to get restful sleep.

The sleep apnea drops to subclinical status as if by magic. His snoring impacted on Charlotte's rest as well; now that the apnea has eased, they're sleeping in the same room again.

It is misplaced gratitude that compels David to wire me box seats for my long-suffering Mets, tickets that probably should have gone to the nutritionist. (However, she's a Yankees fan. In order to spare her the bother of tossing the tickets in the trash, I keep them.) David further shocks Charlotte by joining a meditation class. With his mind clearer, he finds that he is now working more efficiently than ever. It doesn't escape his notice that he is also enjoying his non-work life, and time with his wife, more than he has in years.

"It's all win-win," he says, his grin displaying that endearing gap between his front teeth.

My Mets, who are on their annual downward spiral, lose the game for which David bought me tickets. If that's one reality I can't remake, I can choose to remain absurdly hopeful, nonetheless.

Chapter 5

Case of the Runaway Bride (Meridian Tapping)

With his rakish, semi-automatic grin, easy manner and athletic build, Darrell, 31, would seem to have it all. But two weeks before their destination wedding, his fiancée unceremoniously dumped him. The shock has sparked sleeplessness, anxiety, depression, and loss of appetite.

"Been a rough five weeks." Darrell looks down at his Dr Martens. "Never had a problem sleeping," he says. "But then, no one ever …" At this point, Darrell becomes silent.

"It's called Acute Insomnia. It might be triggered by sudden loss, a relationship ending, or a change of home or job." In most cases, it eases when a period of grieving has run its course. At other times, as in the case with Darrell, it may linger.

Even now, Darrell blames himself for the breakup.

"I think I need an exorcist." He sounds as if he was only half-joking.

"Let's try Meridian Tapping instead."

Many of the tools in Rewired stem from older systems of medicine. Progressive Muscle Relaxation is rooted in Yoga. Neuro-Linguistic Programming (NLP) is an offshoot of trance work, a four thousand year-old system from Egypt. Acupressure is rooted in therapy from ancient China. In contrast, Meridian Balancing came of age in the 1980's, or roughly mid-period Flock of Seagulls era. But when we stack its component parts — acupressure and NLP — you'd have seven thousand years of knowledge compressed into a deceptively simple protocol that is very good at clearing out old programming.

Exercise 6: Meridian Tapping

At first blush, this audacious meld of acupressure and Neuro-Linguistic Programming might seem like a gimmick, or even a child's game. I assure you, neither one is the case. Its most vocal supporter, Gary Craig, worked with it, expanded its scope and then renamed it Emotional Freedom Technique (EFT). The system, he says, clears old trauma by combining touch with verbal desensitization.

In Craig's view, it is an "electrical malfunction" that is at the root of negative emotional states. It's not a memory of a past experience that causes trauma, so much as a disruption in the body's energy system that takes place after the memory. He likens the energy flowing through our body to that of a TV set. If you were to take off the back of your TV set and probe through its electronics with a metal screwdriver, you'd get a short circuit. The picture and sound would become erratic and the TV would exhibit its version of a "negative emotion."

Similarly, a trauma — real or perceived — can create an internal short-circuiting effect. In theory, by tapping on specific points and changing what we say, we reboot both body and mind. Over the years, I've found Tapping to be effective enough to warrant its inclusion here.

The sequence entails tapping points on the head and body while making a declarative statement on the ongoing problem. Tap gently three or four times per point, and then

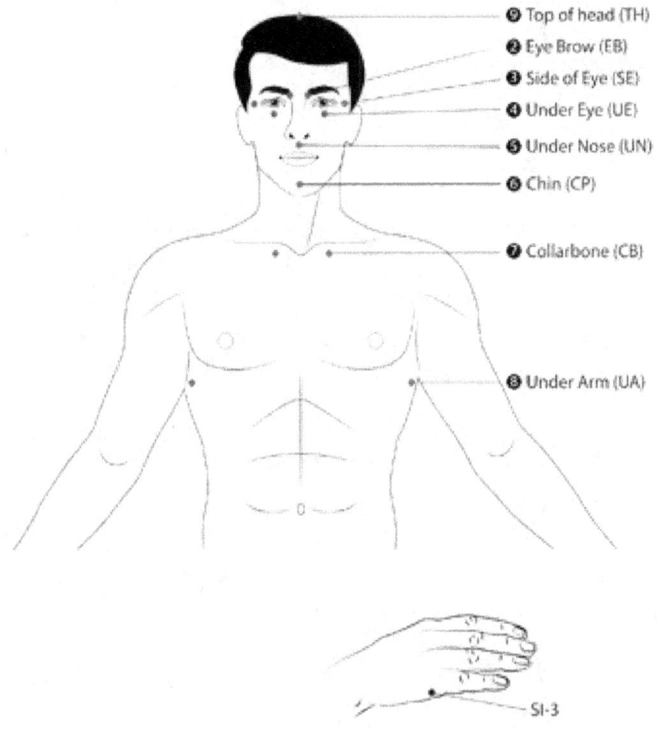

Tapping, Round 1

1. Establish a negative feeling or sensation that you wish to get rid of. As an example, we can state: "I'm anxious that I can't sleep." Your goal is to clear away the negative feeling.

2. Ask yourself, "Where in my body do I experience the feeling?" It might take a moment to locate it. Let's say for now that it's like a tight, hard fist in the pit of your stomach.

3. On a scale of 1 to 10 (with ten being awful), ask yourself, "What number am I now?" It's possible that you'll first do this exercise when you feel calm. Even so, close your eyes for a moment, and mentally recall a time when you were in bed—the previous night perhaps—and feeling awful because you were unable to sleep. If you can't call it up, that's okay too.

But let's say you've managed to recreate the "bad feeling". Now raise the intensity level up to an eight or nine. In a moment you'll start Tapping on the feeling to lessen its impact.

Create a sort of story, subtly changing the words as you go. State how you feel now, and then slowly shift the phrases to express the desired state. Write it out as an arc. Start with a negative state (I feel like crap; can't sleep; I'm angry) and slowly reframe it to express the way you'd prefer to feel.

If you go to Part III, in "Other Voices, Other Modules, you will find various examples of how I used Meridian Tapping.

Use one of those as a template or create your own arc from among them.

Darrel stands facing me while I demonstrate for him the nine points we will tap on.

"Where in your body is the grief?" I begin.

"Been trying to avoid that shite."

"Is it working for you?"

"Not even a little."

"Take a moment to briefly think about the breakup. Where's the feeling in your body?" As he shifts his weight uneasily, I say, "Is it in your belly, your chest, in your head? Let yourself bring it up."

"Laura," he says at last, "is a rock in my chest."

As he recalls the breakup, he is able to raise his level of discomfort, from a "five" to an "eight." For our purposes, I'll use "Relationship's over." Substitute your problem where the italics now sit. Using the three middle fingers of one hand, begin tapping the other hand.

1. Tap the Karate point [S.I point]: "I feel bad over the relationship ending, and I accept myself."

2. Tap the Eyebrow point [EB] "Relationship's over and I can't sleep."

3. Temple point [T] (Rephrase the bad feeling): "Feel like crap."

4. Under-Eye point [UE]: (Dilute its strength): "Sometimes feel like crap. Relationship."

5. Under nose [UN]: Introduce self-care: "Relationship's done. Totally accept myself."

6. Chin [C]: Combine the phrases: "Depressed, felt bad, accept myself."

7. Collarbone point [CB]: (it's universal, natural): "Accept myself. I'm only human. I'm allowed to feel bad, I'm allowed to sleep."

8. Under arm [UA]: (you can feel good) Shift time frame to diminish an undesired emotional state: "I've *felt* depressed. Feeling okay. Letting go of her, and totally accept myself."

9. Top of head [TOH] (Introduce desired state/self-acceptance): "I can move on, love myself."

Next, connect the left/right hemispheres of the brain. Bring your hands down. Intertwine them so your right hand is on the left, and your left hand on your right. Take a deep breath and bring your hands up to your chest. Hold the breath for three seconds. As you exhale, shake out your body as if you were shaking water from your body.

"What number are you at now?" I ask Darrell.

"Four?"

"Try and raise it back up to a nine."

"I can't. It's maybe a soft six?"

In the next round we add stronger emotions into the mix.

Tapping, Round 2

1. "Even though I sometimes feel sad, I completely accept myself." Repeat this several times. Each time you do so, gently tap the K (Karate) point three times.

2. Eyebrow point [EB] Source: "Done with that person, can't sleep."

3. Temple point [T] Rephrase: "Sleep sucks right now."

4. Under-Eye point [UE]: Dilute: "Sometimes sad, sometimes feel awesome."

5. Under nose [UN]: Introduce self-care: "Screw her, totally accept myself."

6. Chin [C]: Combine phrases: "Sometimes can't sleep, completely accept myself."

7. Collarbone point [CB]: "I'm only human. It's okay to feel bad, it's okay to sleep."

8. Under arm [UA]: Shift time frame to weaken the unwanted state. "I've felt bad. Feeling okay. Letting go, feeling strong and totally accept myself."

9. Top of head [TH]: Desired state and self-acceptance: "I can sleep, I love myself."

Intertwine your hands left over right, raise them to your chest, take a deep breath and hold it for three seconds. As you exhale, shake out your arms, and then shake out your body.

When I ask him to bring up the "bad feeling" again, he says, "I can't".

When I next see Darrell, a scowl has eclipsed the previous week's damaged charm. While I'm glad he is in touch with his feelings, I'm almost afraid to ask how he is doing.

"I'm pissed off."

"And how's the sleep going?"

"Messed up. That's how angry I am."

"You want to hang on to the anger?" I am aware that I am treading on thin ice.

"Angry feels … good right now. Like picking at a scab good. I guess I just want to forget about her, or at least not hang on any longer than I … have to."

I'll step back from discussing Darrell for a moment, and instead speak with you, the reader.

Let's postulate that you are upset by what someone said or did. You've been wronged. It's eating you up and keeping you up. Here's the problem: the guilty party has probably moved on. The only person stuck inside of that toxic dumpsite … is you. We know that wounds heal with time, but sometimes that's the long way around. Maybe you'd rather exit the dumpsite now. If so, then Meridian Tapping can help.

Darrell Taps on Anger

(K) "Angry at _________ and totally accept myself."

(EB) "Angry as hell …"

(T) "Totally accept myself…"

(UE) "Really pissed off … Accept"

(UN) "Getting _____ out of my brain. Love myself."

(C) "I'm allowed to get free of _____, accept myself."

(CB) "I'm powerful, Accept."

(UA) "Letting go of old toxins, letting go."

(TOH) "Letting go. Accept myself."

Darrell is talking with a therapist, something he might not have done had the wedding gone ahead as planned. "She's my consolation prize," he tells me, the hint of a smile on his otherwise long face.

That said, the aftershock affected Darrell's appetite; he has lost fifteen pounds, weight he can ill afford to lose. I have him massage acupoint Stomach 36 (ST36, Zu San Li or Leg Three Miles). ST36 helps mitigate digestive problems including gastric pain, appetite, vomiting, abdominal distention, diarrhea, and constipation while easing insomnia, heart palpitations, shortness of breath, dizziness, and anxiety.

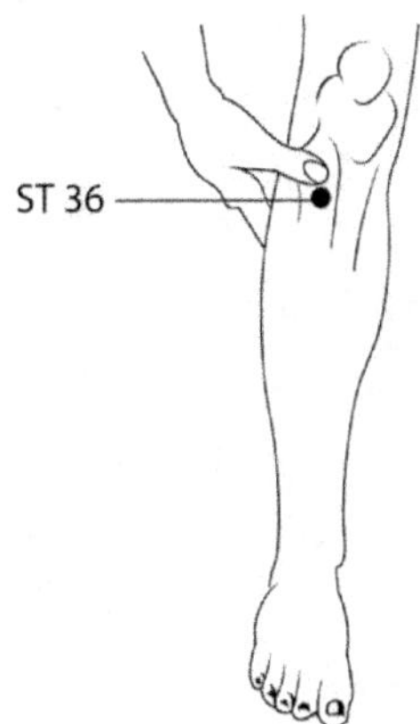

The acupoint sits on the outer part of the leg, below the knee. Place four fingers just below your kneecap. It's at the edge of your pinky, a finger's breadth on the outside your shinbone. Many who would know consider ST36). to be the most powerful acupoint on the body, and as a result massage or use controlled heat on that point daily to increase longevity.

As Darrell finds sleep again, his appetite also returns — and in more ways than one.

"Maybe I'm a glutton," he says sheepishly, "but I just went on three dating sites."

"Three? I guess you're ready?" Suddenly I have become a dating guru.

"Only one way to find out." Darrell turns the full force of his pearly whites my way.

"Full steam ahead! Oh, and you might consider doing Remake Your Day."

"Why would I do that?"

"To rewire your neural circuits for the ending you want. The good ending, this time."

Online dating proves to be an eye opener for Darrell. His damaged ego was in need of some TLC, and the rollicking online forum has clearly provided it for him, in spades.

As he heads out after an acupuncture session, he pauses at the door. I wait.

"Did I mention that Laura contacted me?"

"Really?" In some circles this is called a doorknob confession. "How did she...?"

'On a dating site. Strangest thing." He shrugs. "I knew it was too late for us."

"What tipped you off?"

"When I Remade my Day? She wasn't anywhere in it."

We'll return to Meridian Tapping time and again; this tool is that effective. If you would like more information on this system, search for EFT online for helpful videos on different sorts of issues.

Chapter 6:

Progressive Muscle Relaxation

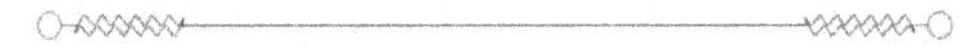

Luis and Rebound Insomnia

Luis, 41, a handyman at a tony 5th Avenue address, hurt his back on the job. The pain is sharp and worse at night, making sleep difficult. This thin Honduran-born man has bottomless eyes that seem to soak in worry.

"Doctor gave me a muscle relaxer." He unconsciously massages his lower back. "Works good at first and I can sleep. Then it wears off and I wake up."

Rebound Insomnia is defined by being wakened when medication (or alcohol) wears off. In Luis's case, the medication is for his pain, which is severe. To complicate matters, he has a second child on the way, and fear of being fired from his job ignites barely-latent anxiety, this despite being a card-carrying member of a union; everyone has heard about people being deported while awaiting citizenship.

Luis has resigned himself to losing it all and then being deported back to Honduras. He tells me this as he gets off the table and tries stretching. That's when he realizes that his frozen, painful low back has released by some eighty percent. Luis leaves my office light of heart and with renewed hope.

But before he leaves, I explain to him that pain often returns, whether from muscle memory or from renewed strain. Repeated treatment is warranted. He nods his head, saying yes, yes, doctor Dan, I will be in touch. In his mind, he is cured, and the pin man is history.

There are times when I am sorry that I'm right. This is one such time. Five days after I last see Luis, he is back looking more disheartened than when he first came in.

As Luis signs on for a series of acupuncture treatments, he asks me how he can help himself. I gladly show him a stretching exercise, along with several acupoints that he, or his wife, can use for massage.

One such point is called Triple Warmer 3 (TW3). While it's classically used more for headache, tinnitus, and sore throat, TW3 also is effective for low back pain.

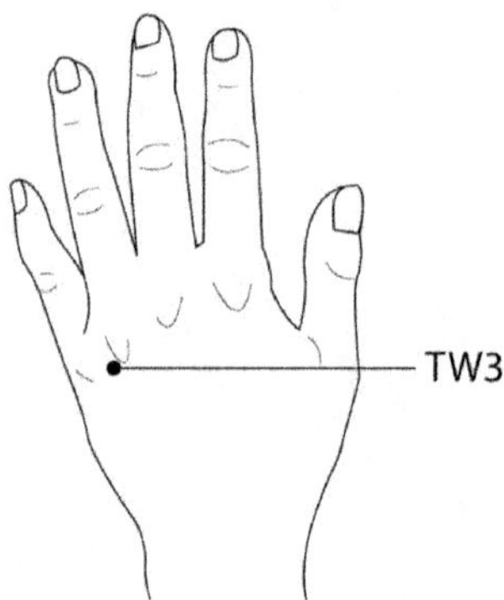

When the fist is clenched, the point is on the back of the hand between the fourth and fifth metacarpal bones, in the depression. (See illustration). Locate a spot that you find to be "ouchy" and massage it for two minutes.

Relax the Muscles, Relax the Mind

Progressive Muscle Relaxation, or PMR, is an exercise that coaches and therapists teach their clients to relax the body and mind.

"PMR brings oxygen to the body while flushing out toxins," I tell Luis, who often looks dubious about anything I tell him. "It might take ten, fifteen minutes at first, then it gets easier."

Find a quiet place where you won't be disturbed. This might be at home in a recliner, or in nature — anywhere with minimal distractions, and with no cellphone, computer, kids, or spouses about. You can lie down, or not. Wear loose, comfortable clothing, and remove your shoes.

We will target fourteen muscle groups, one area at a time. For instance, you can focus on the muscles of your left hand. Take a breath, and as you inhale, squeeze the muscles for ten seconds. Really feel the tension. Make the muscle tension deliberate, yet gentle. As you exhale, relax the muscles. Hold the relaxed state for about ten seconds, then move on to the next muscle group. After you've completed all of the muscle groups, notice how you feel.

Exercise 7: Progressive Muscle Relaxation

You can listen to a recording of Progressive Muscle Relaxation at rewiredforsleep.com/the-deeper-levels.

The best strategy is to start at your feet and slowly move your way upward. For example:

1. Toes: Curl the toes of your left foot without tensing your legs. Hold them for five seconds, counting slowly. Release them and relax. Count to ten, keeping your toes relaxed.

2. Feet and toes: Curl your toes and foot for five seconds, then relax.

3. Calf muscle: Flex your left calf muscle by pulling your toes toward you.

4. Thigh: Contract your left thigh muscles tightly. Hold that for about ten seconds, then relax for ten seconds. (Repeat on the right side.)

5. Left hand: Clench your fist for five seconds, then relax it.

6. Left arm: Tighten your biceps by drawing your forearm up toward your shoulder and making a muscle, while clenching the fist. (Repeat on right side.)

7. Buttocks: Tense and squeeze your buttocks together for ten seconds. Relax for ten seconds and feel yourself releasing the tension.

8. Stomach: Tighten your abdominal muscles by pulling in your stomach for ten seconds. Relax and fully release your stomach muscles for ten seconds.

9. Chest: Take a long, deep breath, tighten your chest muscles, and hold for ten seconds. Exhale and relax for ten seconds, breathing comfortably.

10. Neck: Tighten your neck muscles for ten seconds, then relax for ten seconds.

11. Shoulders: Raise your shoulders up, hold that for ten seconds, then relax them for ten seconds. Do not push this pose if you have an injury.

12. Jaw: Clench then unclench your jaw, then open your mouth wide to stretch out.

13. Eyes: Clench your eyelids tightly shut, then relax them. Open them widely for ten seconds, then relax them for ten seconds.

14. Forehead: Raise your eyebrows, then relax them.

Note: There are many relaxation MP3s for sale that will take you through a similar sort of progressive muscle relaxation. You can find a recording at https://rewiredforsleep.com/the-deeper-levels. There is also a free MP3 available for download to Rewired Sanctuary members. Luis' Honduran mother was a curandera, a wise woman, so he is familiar with liniments like Po Sum On oil.

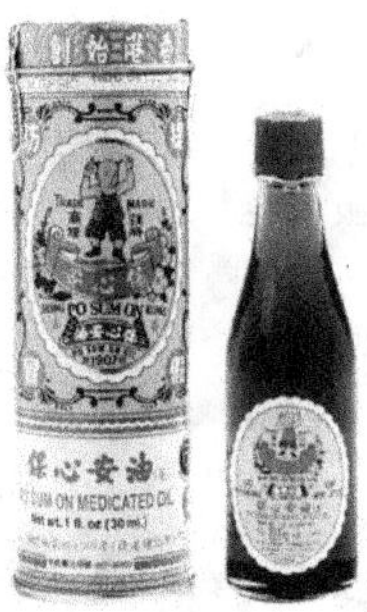

At night, his wife gently rubs it into his tight muscles in circular fashion. With its contents of menthol, skullcap root, Chinese licorice, cinnamon oil, dragon's blood resin, peppermint oil, and tea oil it warms the muscles, improves circulation and relieves pain. Six acupuncture sessions later, Luis is ninety percent pain-free, and he can once more provide for his family. The anxiety he was experiencing around their safety has eased, and he is sleeping better as a result. That said, he still wakes briefly at 2:45

a.m., which he chalks up to living within the vibrating gemstone that is New York City. I don't for a moment doubt that he's right.

I record for him a guided visualization, "Honduran Rainforest" (find it in Extra Mile 1.5).

Luis now is now implementing greater self-care. He listens to the recording when he has the time to do so, uses the tools, when he can, and vows to return for treatment should the pain return.

Alicia, his wife, who has been suffering with pregnancy-related nausea, along with fierce low back pain that radiates down to her buttocks*, becomes a patient.

*Bonus point: Gallbladder 30.

Sciatic pain can leave us tossing and turning at night in an effort to find a comfortable sleeping position. GB30, which can help relieve muscle-based sciatic pain, is found near the center of the buttocks one third to halfway between the hip joint and the tip of the coccyx. Apply pressure with your thumb or index finger until you feel a dull, achy soreness.

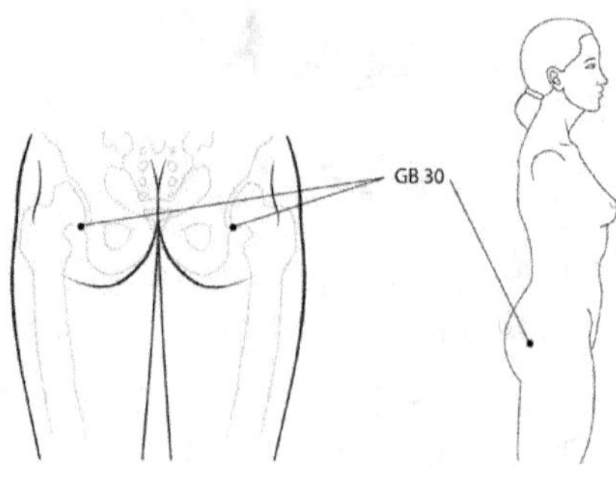

Hold it for thirty seconds. You'll also be able to apply warmth in the form of a Tiger Warmer (we'll discuss that soon).

Chapter 7:

The Case for the Elastic Brain

Now that we're juggling Chinese medicine and Neuro-Linguistic Programming, let's add to the mix physics, neuroscience, and even a touch of linguistics. We'll have use for them all.

The Pauli Exclusion Principle

The Pauli Exclusion Principle is the quantum mechanical principle which states that two or more identical fermions (particles with half-integer spin) cannot occupy the same state simultaneously. This effect is partly responsible for the more simple observation that two solid objects cannot be in the same place at the same time. On an experiential level, this law of physics holds true for the mind as well: your brain can't think two different thoughts simultaneously. You can imagine fear or tranquility, but you can't conjure fear and tranquility in the same instant any more than two electrons can occupy the same physical space. Your brain tends to latch on to the first thought it "sees," and then runs with it. Right now, it's usually the one that's disruptive to sleep.

There is also this:

Neurons That Fire Together ...

Psychologist Donald Hebb put it this way: "Neurons that fire together, wire together." This axiom is a roadmap for rewiring the brain. For neurons to build connections to other neurons, one neuron needs to be firing at the same time another neuron is firing. When neurons fire together, a connection between them is strengthened.

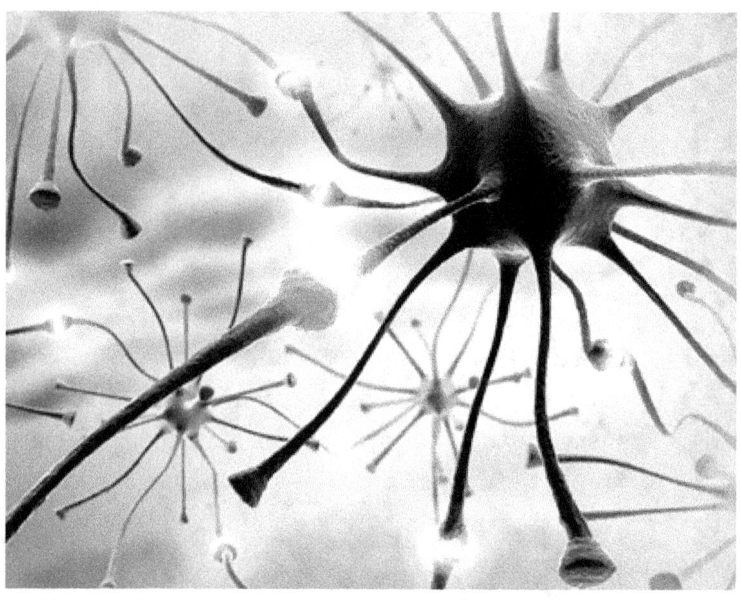

After a while, activating one neuron also activates the other one. As more neurons connect to fire together, this creates a whole set of connected neurons, which then leads the formation of new circuits. These new circuits, called neural networks, result in changes in the brain or learning.

Your past experience dictates how your specific brain circuitry develops. You might associate cigars with a beloved grandfather, while another person will smell a cigar and recall dank horserace parlors. Simply recalling your first day in school can activate new neural circuits. So can a change in behavior, such as practicing the violin. Even the act of imagining a particular behavior, like practicing scales on the violin causes changes in neural circuitry.

In fact, the new science of Neuroplasticity tells us that the ability to create new neurons, the building blocks of change is high up on the brain's list of chores.

Neuroplasticity

In Soft-Wired: How the New Science of Brain Plasticity Can Change Your Life, Dr. Michael Merzenich lays out how change occurs in the brain:

1. If the brain is ready for change, change will happen.

2. The greater the motivation to change, the bigger the brain change.

3. The more something is practiced, the more neurons make connections to enhance the change and include all elements of the experience (sensory information, movement, cognitive patterns).

4. Initial changes are temporary. Only if your brain judges that the outcome is good, is it made permanent.

5. The brain is changed by internal mental rehearsal in the same ways, and involving precisely the same processes, that control changes achieved through interactions with the external world.

6. As you learn a new skill, your brain remembers the successful attempts, while discarding the failed ones. Then, it makes incremental adjustments to make progressive improvements.

We can now see why Remake Your Day, or similar exercise, can benefit the psyche.

A Brief History of Anxiety and Depression

We tend to think of anxiety and depression as purely modern phenomena. Claudius Galen personal physician to Marcus Aurelius in the second century A.D., described a patient with melancholic delusions, who feared that Atlas would get tired and drop the world.

Other patients of Galen experienced "scarce, turbulent, and interrupted sleep, palpitations, vertigo … sadness, anxiety, diffidence, and belief of being persecuted, of being possessed by a demon, hated by the gods …" Galen treated depression and anxiety using his own patent recipes of plantains, mandrake, linden flowers, opium, and arugula.

Exercise 8: Autogenic Training

We all want control over our own body. When we sense that it's failing us, it's easy for negative self-talk to gain a foothold in the mind. "Insomnia is controlling my body; stress is controlling me …" Autogenic Training helps us fight back against self-talk.

Autogenic Training (AT) was invented in 1932 by one Dr. Schultz, a German cardiologist. It is my understanding that he created AT after growing tired of watching his patients die. His goal in formulating this program was so his patients could learn to regulate their own blood pressure and heart rate. We can only imagine how many people with cardiac problems could be helped if they were taught AT. You'll find a recording for Autogenic Training at https://rewiredforsleep.com/the-deeper-levels. Begin with a bit of Chinese medicine. Massage Yintang and Under 3rd Toe twenty-four times in each direction, while taking deep breaths. Notice how the diagrams almost mirror one another.

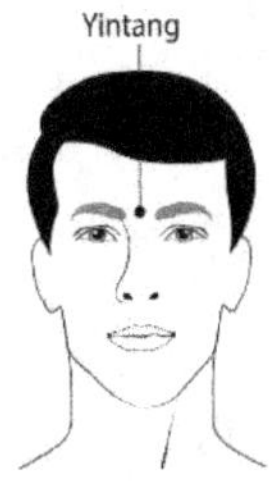

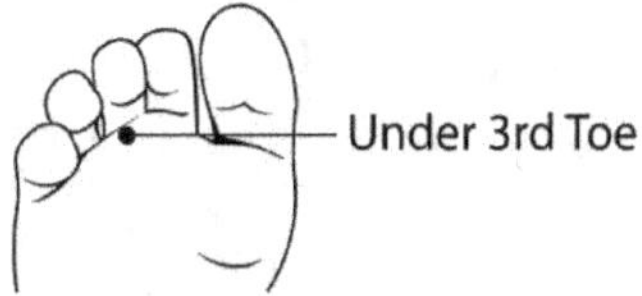

Autogenic Training I

You can listen to a recording of Autogenic Training at https://rewiredforsleep.com/the-deeper-levels

Do the exercise while seated, or lying down, whichever you prefer. Take in a breath and close your eyes. As you breathe in and breathe out, scan your body. If you're carrying tension, breathe into the areas or tension, be it your neck, your back, and so on. As you breathe, focus on this time that you've set aside to increase your control over your body, calmly and effortlessly. Let your hands rest on your lap and uncross your feet. With each long breath out, allow yourself to relax more deeply.

Now focus on your hands. Notice how your hands are relaxed, as they rest on your lap. And now, with each breath, your hands can become even more relaxed. Once you focus on your relaxed hands, notice how, when hands are truly relaxed, they're very heavy. In fact, as you notice your relaxed hands you can even say to yourself, out loud or in your own mind, "My hands are heavy. My hands are heavy." Go ahead and say that, either aloud or in your own mind. "My hands are heavy. My hands are heavy."

Allow your hands to feel that sense of heaviness, as you breathe in, and breathe out.

Think of the word warmth, and as you focus on your heavy hands say to yourself, "My hands are warm. My hands are warm." And as you say that to yourself, notice the sensation of warmth in those hands. Actually say to yourself, "My hands are warm. My hands are warm." Notice the sensation of warmth.

As you breathe in, and breathe out, say to yourself, "My hands are warm and heavy. My hands are warm and heavy." Now, continue to breathe in, and breathe out, with each breath doubling that sensation of relaxation, enjoying this time with yourself. Now open the eyes. Take in a deep breath, fill the lungs with oxygen and reorient back into the room. [Find Autogenic Training II in The Extra Mile 1.5]

Now let's apply the Pauli Exclusion Principle to beliefs about sleep. We'll keep the choices binary-simple: "I can't sleep" or "I control my mind." The laws of physics will apply either way, so you may as well choose the one that you prefer. And if you have decided that you have no choice in your beliefs, that too is a reality that's available for change. In fact, changing our reality is often as easy as changing the words we use.

Exercise 9: Use Your Words About Sleep Wisely.

The sleepless mind is like having an overactive child — not your own — in your mind, posing endless, useless questions.

Maybe you know the sort that I'm referring to: "What's wrong with me that I can't _________?" Or, "Why didn't I _________when I had the chance?"

Self-talk that is negative in nature would seem to be part of the human condition. Some people are infrequent visitors to that dark place; others pretty much live there. The dual problem with this inquisition-style self-talk is that it's unproductive, and it spikes chemicals that kill sleep.

Monitor your inner monologue. Start shifting the words you use — and the suppositions behind them. In this way we can begin to dismantle a negative mental loop, replacing it with one that serves our needs. In the past we have all used words or phrases that don't serve us. These in particular are ripe for substitution:

OLD	REPLACE WITH
I always (wake too early)	At times (as in, 'at times I wake up at 3 am'
Must, Should	Can, Might (I might open today's mail, I can sleep tonight)
Don't ever	Sometimes (I sometimes let go of this lingering pain)
Never	Sometimes (I sometimes sleep well)
My .... (illness)	The old...... (illness)
I am a(n) .... (insomniac)	I've experienced..... (sleep issues)

How do you usually describe your sleep issue?

Let's say you want to relegate the sleep issue to the past, or to reframe it as a state that you're moving through?

How might that sound, look, or feel like to you?

How do you usually describe your sleep issue?

Let's say you want to relegate the sleep issue to the past, or to reframe it as a state that you're moving through?

How might that sound, look, or feel like to you?

Affirmations, and the Power of Words

If you've ever started a diet but quit five days later, begun writing your memoirs but then gave up, or tried to learn a language, then you know that follow-through can be hard. Our tendency is to blame our "failure" on a lack of will power. That's not the real problem. Only ten percent of mental activity resides in the conscious mind, while the other ninety percent sits in the subconscious. Imagine trying to lift an eighty-pound weight using ten percent of your muscles, and that seeming collapse of will power may be seen in a new light.

Now, imagine being able to access even thirty percent of the potential that's in your unconscious mind, and you'll get a sense of your own untapped capabilities. Of course, we all would like to have more control of our mind, but what does that have to do with sleep? Affirmations are a strong vehicle for accessing sleep-related inner reserves.

You may think of an affirmation as a contract that we make between our subconscious mind, our self, and the world. This is no new age phenomenon. A core tenet in Eastern thinking, *Sankalpa* is a Sanskrit word meaning resolve, or intention. In fact, history is thick with positive thought. In the 1800's, a French pharmacist, Emile Coue, recognized the power of the subconscious mind to affect inner change. With each prescription he gave out, he included a positive note. "I have never cured anyone in my life," he would say, "I just show people how they can cure themselves." This simple tenet is at the core of a great deal of healing work.

When you are ready to make a positive change, the first step is to state your intention aloud and in the present tense. "I sleep soundly" holds more weight for the unconscious mind than "I'm going to sleep well." Other examples of affirmations include:

- I have an unlimited capacity to sleep well.

- I am waking with more energy every day.

- My self-confidence is increasing by leaps and bounds.

- At the end of the day, I feel sleepy.

- I sleep beautifully through the night.

- The stress that others feel bounces right off me.

- I make any change I want easily and effortlessly.

- By forgiving all those who hurt me, I am free from the prison of resentment.

Use one of these affirmations or create your own. It's best to stick with one or two, and repeat them in your car, while doing the dishes, or any other time. Make your affirmations as bold, delicious, and audacious as you want your life to be. Write one or more affirmations here:

Tony Robbins, the motivational speaker, has talked about his own process of self-growth. As an overweight, teen-age pizza delivery boy, he'd drive his car with the windows rolled up, passionately yelling his intentions out to the universe. People who were in other cars would see some apparently crazed kid screaming his head off.

But with every pizza Tony delivered, he was slowly rewiring his brain to become the motivational guru he is now. Perhaps you can achieve similar results doing what Tony did; I believe he'd say there are easier paths to get there, including affirmation work and guided visualization.

We'll return to the topic of affirmations in the Betty E. self-hypnosis section, where there is context for their use. For now, consider how you might rewire your circuits to work the way you'd want them to.

Chapter 7: The Case for the Elastic Brain

Chapter 8:

Chinese Medicine, and Ancient Tattoos

Ötzi Gets Some Ink

Ever since a psychiatrist prescribed Adderall to manage Brody's anxiety, the tall, jangly 13-year old has had trouble sleeping. He sits across from me in pricey high tops, with Emily, his mom, at his side. Emily blames Adderall — and in private, her divorce — for Brody's sleep problems. What worries her even more is that Brody's asthma, which had been dormant, is once more acting up.

> "I'm hoping acupuncture can help him sleep," she tells me. "I'd be thrilled if you could somehow lower his Adderall dosage as well. I feel horrible for letting them talk me into giving it to him."

L-Theanine, along with herbs such as Kava can help patients with ADHD. I assure Emily and Brody that side effects from the combination are rare, and mother and son are on board with this program.

A verbally expressive young man, Brody shares with me his plan to explore the Antarctic. He's also highly curious, and the topic of acupuncture is not immune from his probing mind.

> "I read about Ötzi," he says. "The five-thousand-year-old guy found in ice in the alps, with tats they think were acupuncture points? I thought my crew invented it." That he's of Chinese-

American descent would be irrelevant but for the charming, unbridled tone of sheer pride in his young voice.

"Your crew was brilliant at observing the body," I reply, "then using those observations to create a comprehensive system of medicine. As for Ötzi, the tats served as a marker for him. If he got sick while traveling, he could press, or massage those spots, and thus help himself."

"How'd they know where how to ink him?"

"A shaman or Village elder would have known." My mind scrolls back to Doña Regina. Grandmother must surely have been part of a lineage of wise women healers.

The Inner Thermostat

"What does it mean if I kick my covers off at night?" Brody is warming to the topic.

"Sleep is dependent on our state of the mind. If we're calm, we sleep well. But if the body's thermostat malfunctions, heat rises to disturb the mind, and we can't sleep."

"How do I reset it?"

"Certain acupoints can help. For instance, there is a point on the bottom of the foot that eases insomnia, palpitations, anxiety, and night sweats." I doubt Brody would care that it also eases hot flashes and poor memory. (Note: for hot flashes, see Ginger Rogers and the Hot Flash).

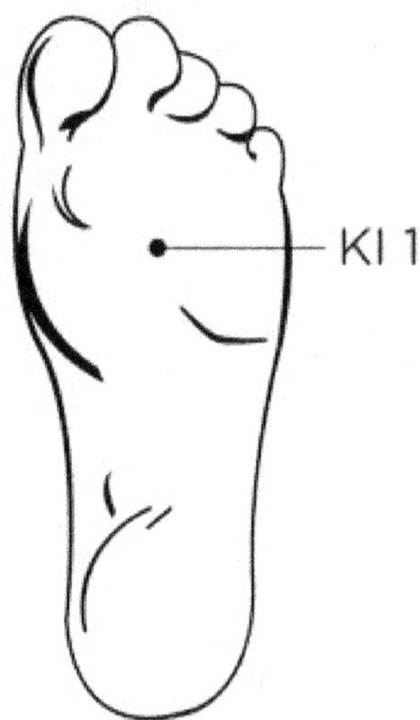

It's called Kidney 1 (KI1 Yongquan, or Gushing Spring) and is found on the sole, in the depression about 1/3 down the length of the foot and directly between the 2nd and 3rd toes. It may or may not feel achy to the touch.

"So I press it," says Brody, "and my brain cools down, just like that?"

"It's not a magic button. Think of the points as gentle reminders, nudging the body toward a state of internal balance. Press around Kidney 1, and massage the most 'ouchy' area twenty-four times, first clockwise then counter-clockwise."

"I read that in China there are whole libraries on this medicine," he says, probing the bottom of his foot with his thumbs. "How does it actually work?"

"I could tell you how acupuncture eases muscle tension, which increases oxygen to the cells and moves toxins out of the body, or how it releases lymph to improve immune function. But since the science is rooted in nature, I'll use the image of a river to explain it. Normally, water flows without being blocked or spilling onto its banks. Animal and plant life thrive there. It's a healthy river. This also describes a body and mind when it's healthy. Now, imagine that same river but with a dam across the middle of it. One side has nowhere to go so it overflows its banks, while the other side is a stagnant pool with moldy leaves and twigs. This describes a state of poor health. How would we make that river healthy again?"

"You've got to unblock those dams. How do you know where to find them?"

"We've got a map. You see, Chinese medicine tells us the body's got fourteen circuits, or meridians, coursing through it. These meridians transport blood, nutrients, and a substance called Qi. When a blockage impedes that flow, we get pain, inflammation … and messy sleep. By mentally overlaying our map onto the body, we know where to place pins to release blockage."

"To keep it all moving," Brody says. "But what is Qi?"

"Think of it as energy moving in the body." Why try and explain to him that some consider Qi to be oxygen, while others see it as vital life force, or even its own unique substance. That said, enough people have experienced Qi to describe its workings in minute detail: where it begins, where it travels in the body, and even what type of Qi it is.

 "Explain to me why I press my ankle if I want to get rid of a headache?"

"Again, think circuits. If you wanted to turn on an overhead light, you'd flip a wall switch instead of climbing a ladder to screw in the bulb. Same thing with the body. It's got endless switches that turn on the overhead light we call the human brain."

Since Brody has asthma, and he breathes from his chest rather than from his belly, I give mother and son a mini-seminar on abdominal breathing. Emily vows to monitor Brody's breathing from hereon in. This is also a good time to discuss diet. If the link between Brody's ADHD and his consumption of soda and sugary cereal had not been clear to Emily before, at least she is now on board with weaning him off sugar.

What's more, Brody is now sleeping with his head at the foot of his bed. This is not so strange, really. By changing positions, he has displaced what had become an antagonistic relationship with his bed. This simple rewiring process meshes with the 7-Day Neuroplasticity Challenge from week three of the 28-Day Repair Program. That said, Brody dislikes doing the Five, Five, and Five Exercise and we negotiate that down to a "Two, Two, and Two". He promises to work his way up from there.

After eight sessions over ten weeks, Brody is asleep earlier than he had been, waking only briefly at 2:00 a.m. Emily is thrilled that he has stopped wheezing and no longer needs the inhaler.

"He seems more focused," she comments. "Less all over the place."

Financial considerations are such that we've put further treatment on hold for now. But his dependence on Adderall is down by two thirds. Emily emailed me that he appears poised to stop using it altogether. His progress doesn't surprise me, really.

In truth, it would not shock me if one day he made his way to his beloved Antarctic.

Chapter 9:

How I Learned to Stop Worrying and Love

Qi Gong

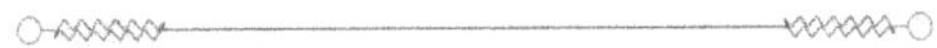

Hearing the Voice Within.

Among those of us who landed in acupuncture college, a portion were newbies, myself included. My deer-in-the-headlights crew included a former filmmaker, a computer nerd, a graphics artist, and a publicist. I was a musician. Despite formal training, I'd dived into the post-punk scene and spent the 1980's in New York playing all of the clubs, from the grittiest to the most grand. I'll admit that, even now, it can be comforting to bask in the dim light of my younger, Rebel-Rebel self. But as others who once walked the artistic road will tell you, there came a time when the lifestyle no longer served me any more than the harsh economics of it did. The problem was that I had no backup plan, making a clean break all that much more difficult.

What finally lured me away from that divinely sketchy world was a career that, on its shiny face, seemed both lucrative and exciting. It wasn't long before I discovered that said career was less than as advertised on both counts, and I found myself in a state of confused limbo. The death of my father around that time contributed to a sense of dislocation, and for the first time in my adult life, I was rudderless; adrift. Old fears and childhood anxieties were my new four a.m. companions. Sleep suffered.

Around that time, someone whom we'll call Jim suggested I try Qi Gong (pronounced Chee Gung). Some people view it as martial art, others as a meditation practice. The problem? Jim was my then-landlord. And we were feuding. He was in my apartment because a judge had ordered him to fix my leaky toilet, work that was long overdue. Seeing that I was engrossed in a book on Kundalini Yoga, Jim offered a cogent argument as to why I should try this other system.

At another time, I might have called forth my inner Sid Vicious and told him where he could place his Qi Gong. But just then I was yo-yoing between anxiety and insomnia, and desperate, and perhaps more open to suggestion than I might otherwise have been. Why not give it a try? I had meditated on and off for years, so I felt sure the template would be familiar.

As I did the exercises, their effect on me was impactful. I recovered my lost energy, but equally important, my mind quieted down. I could hear my inner voice telling me not just what I wanted, but what I needed as well. Perhaps you've guessed where this story's going: a year later, I was acupuncture school bound. In truth, I'm grateful to that rascally landlord. And it wasn't only because Jim shone a light onto a path I might not have taken otherwise; he finally fixed that leaky toilet once and for all.

The following exercise is part of Qi Gong, a fully-realized subset of Chinese medicine.

Exercise 10: Six Healing Sounds (Liu Zi Jue)

Anyone who's ever felt the gorgeous thrum of music deep down in their bones knows the power of sound. It's natural then, that the ancients would want to harness it. By "ancients" I am referring to Taoists, a Chinese mystical sect whose philosophy emphasized living in harmony with nature. Much of Asian medicine arose from Taoism ("The Way"), as did its iconic Yin Yang symbol. More than a quaint, tattoo-worthy design, the image is expressive of a view of the universe as a cohesive fusion of seeming opposites.

We first find Six Healing Sounds in a work from the fifth century AD: "On Caring for the Health of the Mind and Prolonging the Life Span," written by Tao Hongling. We know how stressors impact sleep; these exercises help release stressors and send them back out to the ether. You can start clearing out old toxins and building internal Qi from day one. I did.

Breathe in through your nose and exhale through your mouth. Cycle through all six sounds, the first five aloud and the sixth one silently. Note your reaction to each one in your sleep journal, then either continue doing the six (my recommendation) or home in on one or two. Know that you are working with powerful emotions, including anger, joy, obsessive thoughts, grief, and fear. In other words, be gentle with yourself.

Liver/Gallbladder (helps control the quality of the blood and supports eyesight)

The liver/gallbladder sound addresses the emotion of anger. Take a deep breath and, with a long, slow exhale, say SHOOOO. Picture your liver surrounded by a bright green color, and fill it with a feeling of pure kindness (The Inner Smile, Extra Mile 1.5, can assist you in visualizing it). This will enhance the positive energy of the liver during Detoxification. Do each exercise six times, with a brief rest in between.

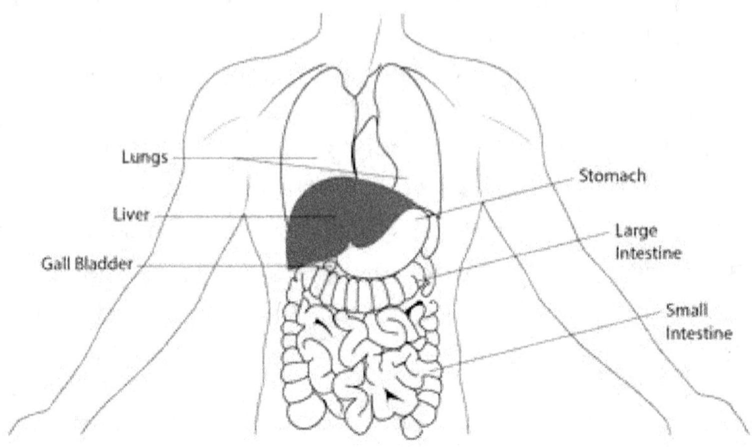

Lungs
Liver
Gall Bladder
Stomach
Large Intestine
Small Intestine

Heart/Small Intestine (controls circulation of the blood)

The emotions associated with the heart are joy, and its flipside, depression. With your mouth open, inhale slowly and then exhale the sound HUHHHHHH (as in "her," without the "r," but in your throat, almost as if you were clearing it). During each resting period, smile into your heart, and picture it surrounded by the color red. Recall a time when you experienced a sense of joy, and then use that image/sound/feeling to enhance the positive energy of the heart.

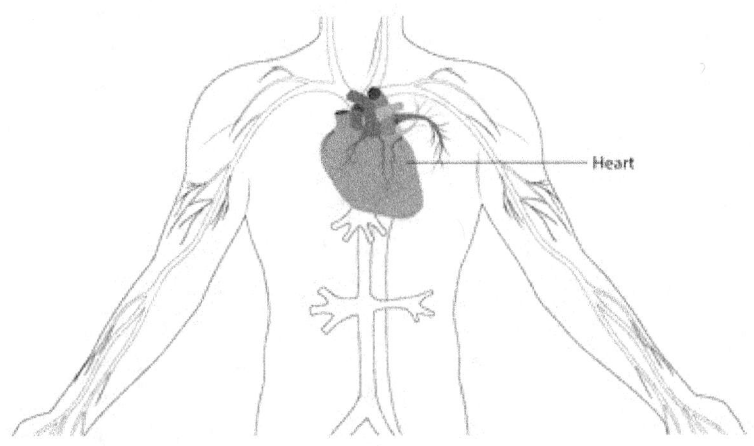

Spleen/Stomach/Pancreas (controls transportation of nutrients)

The emotion associated with the spleen is rumination. If you struggle with OCD, doing this sound may help ease the symptoms. Produce the sound WHOOOOOO from the throat, like the word "who." As you exhale, smile into the spleen and picture it surrounded by a warm, golden yellow color

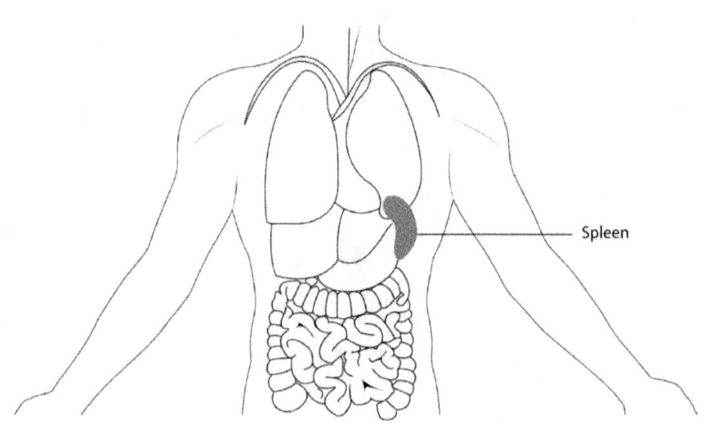

Lungs/Large Intestine (controls the intake of oxygen)

The lung sound addresses grief that hasn't been fully processed and helps to clear it out of the body. Place your tongue behind your closed teeth, and create a SSSSSSSSSS, like the sound of steam coming from a radiator. Picture your lungs surrounded by white light, smile into them and focus on gathering the strength necessary to move forward.

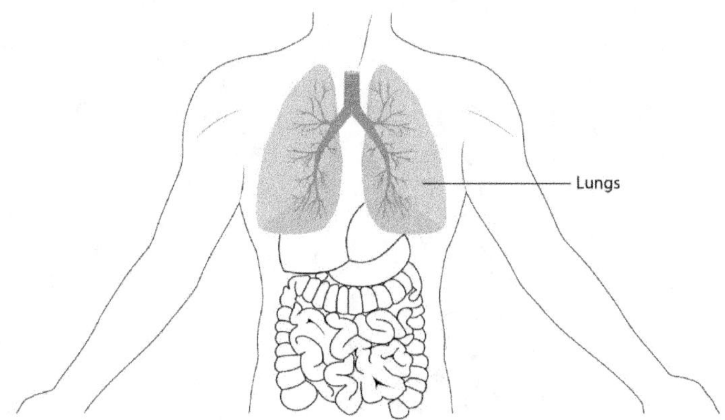

Kidneys/Bladder (Oversees reproduction, urination and memory)

In Chinese medicine, the emotion of fear is part of kidney energy. Since fear and uncertainty often hinder restful sleep, we help our cause by easing unwarranted fear. Start by forming an O with your lips, as if you are preparing to blow out a candle, and with a long, slow exhalation, produce the sound WOOOOOO. The color we associate with the kidneys is blue. Picture your kidneys surrounded by a deep, blue color. As you breathe, send a smile to your kidneys as you visualize inhaling courage and exhaling fear.

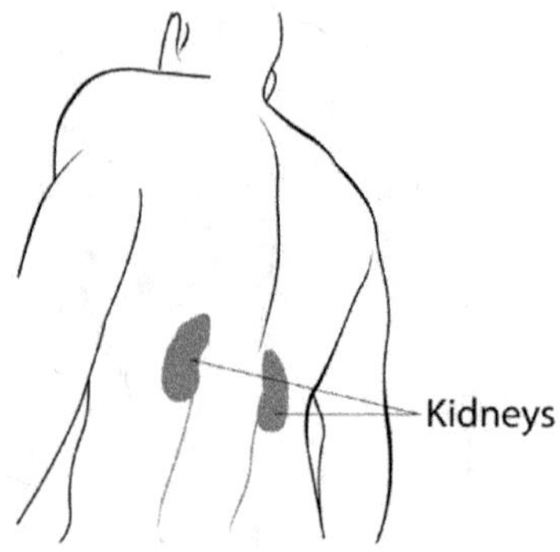

Triple Warmer/Pericardium (harmonizes all the organs)

The Triple Warmer refers to an organ system that harmonizes the energies of the other organs. This exercise is meant to be done while lying down. With your mouth open, slowly exhale as you produce the sound HEEEEEEEEE. Imagine a huge rolling pin flattening your body, from your forehead down to your toes. Aside from harmonizing the other functions, it helps correct any emotional disharmony caused by the stresses of daily life.

Was there one sound in particular that you clicked with?

If the answer is yes, did you get an image (V), was it something about the sound (A) or a feeling in your body (K)? Note that in your sleep journal.

Note: Detoxification often induces what's called a "kill-off reaction." This refers to a natural process whereby a person feels worse before they feel better. If you find that happening, monitor it, but also be aware that you are on your way to taking the next step forward in your health.

Break-In: Spencer Tracy Remakes His Day

Spencer Tracy was a great American film actor from the 20th century. One of his movies, Bad Day at Black Rock called for his character, a one-armed cop, to knock down a man with a single punch. Tracy did the difficult scene in one take. Asked how long he had practiced the balletic move, Tracy said, "I didn't. I just thought about it a lot." Besides being a great actor, he was a master at using visualization to achieve his goals. When you consciously remake your day, you are also creating your own reality.

Chapter 10:

Nutrition Impossible? Sleep-Positive Food

For our purposes, let's agree that everything we do takes us closer to sleep or further from it; toward tranquility or away from it. This idea holds true for what we eat, as well. Support your body with the right food, and it will surely thank you when it's time to sleep. So, what's the "right" food?

Sleep-Positive Food

Healthy fats help provide your body with the necessary building blocks to manufacture sleep hormones. They include coconut oil, organic and pasture-raised meats, eggs, avocado, and butter. Be aware that coconut oil can also act as a stimulant for some people, so monitor how it affects you.

- Eat plenty of high antioxidant foods, as they're important for hormone production and removal of toxins that can impede sleep. Focus on leafy vegetables, high-nutrient fruits, and herbal or green teas — green tea early in the day only, as it contains caffeine.

- It's best to stop eating at least 4 hours before bedtime, and preferably by 6 p.m. every night. Cut back on carbohydrates. Eating protein at this meal will help prepare the body to enter the sleep cycle.

Specific Foods That Encourage Sleep

- Cherry juice – contains melatonin, a sleep-inducing hormone. The tart form is best for sleep.

- Milk – works well warm or cold. The fresh tryptophan in it helps with sleep. Not recommended if you are lactose intolerant. Drinking more than a glass-full in a day is also not suggested.

- Jasmine rice, or a carbohydrate with a high glycemic index metabolizes slowly. This helps your body not work so hard and may calm you. Don't eat them late at night.

- Natural complex carbs. Some experts say no carbs or yogurt near bedtime. Given the sugar content of most yogurt, I tend to agree. There are exceptions, including cereal with low sugar content, barley, quinoa, buckwheat, or plain yogurt with a little fruit or honey.

- Bananas – contain potassium and magnesium; both promote sleep.

- Turkey – think Thanksgiving snooze. It's the tryptophan.

- Sweet potatoes (yams) – a complex-carb superfood that contains sleep-promoting, muscle-relaxing potassium. Other potassium-rich foods include regular potatoes with the skin on, lima beans, papaya and, again, bananas. Eat these foods and relax.

Sleep Deprivation=Hunger

Loss of sleep seriously throws off your body's hormonal profile on multiple levels. Aside from messing with Growth Hormone (GH), it also affects the hormones that regulate your appetite: ghrelin, which is associated with feelings of hunger, and leptin, which is associated with feelings of fullness. Reduced sleep results in an increase in ghrelin and a reduction in leptin levels. If you're trying to restrict your caloric intake, sleep deprivation is telling your brain that it's hungrier than normal. Fatigue makes it even harder to resist your body's hormonal demands. Get that sleep.

Food to Avoid

- When we eat sugar and carbohydrates at night, this creates a blood sugar spike and subsequent crash. It all leads to spotty asleep. As an FYI, if you crave carbs at night, you may have an underlying hormonal problem and should see a professional health practitioner.

- Grains: For the gluten intolerant, grains can cause stress in your body, altering the hormone cycle and impending sleep.

- Vegetable Oils can negatively impact the hormone cycle. Try to stick to olive oil.

- Alcohol might make you sleepy at first but then metabolizes, raising sugar levels to harm the sleep cycle. Just to be a total party pooper, try and avoid alcohol for at least four hours before bed. If you must indulge, drink a glass of water for every glass of alcohol (this helps avoid hangovers).

- Caffeine intake should end six to eight hours before sleep. Chocolate contains caffeine (so sorry), as do energy drinks and most sodas, which are also awash in sugar. Some medications contain caffeine, so read the labels before using them.

- Spicy Foods. Anything spicy is a recipe for sleep disaster. (Side note for menopausal women: spicy foods will also raise the body's temperature, which can impact sleep negatively).

- Anything that is high in saturated fat.

- Tyramine increases the release of norepinephrine, a stress hormone. Food containing high levels of tyramine should be avoided near bedtime. That includes bacon, cheese, chocolate, eggplant, ham, potatoes, sugar, sausage, spinach, and tomatoes.

Journal on which of the above foods you tend to eat. If one of them is on the list that ambushes sleep, make a conscious effort to find a substitute for it. Experiment a bit, and you'll find one.

Write down any item on the list that you'd consider letting go of, or cutting down on, for now:

1.

2.

What we might substitute instead of that food:

1.

2.

> *3 A.M. Munchies? Try Protein.*
>
> *A portion of people who wake up between 2 and 3 a.m. might be hungry (or bored, or anxious) and need to eat. If that describes how you "nosh", prepare beforehand with a small bit of protein, such as a dozen almonds that you can munch on. A drop in insulin has been shown to wake people up, and a bit of protein helps stabilize blood sugar levels, thereby helping you return to sleep.*

Amino Acids That Support Sleep

The following supplements have been chosen for their sleep enhancing abilities. Because we all have unique chemistry, finding the right one for you may involve trial and error on your part.

5-HTP (5-Hydroxtriptophan) This naturally occurring amino acid helps produce serotonin, a chemical messenger that is an important initiator of sleep. Low serotonin levels are associated with depression, anxiety, and sleep disorders. 5-HTP also increases melatonin, which increases stages 3 and 4 of REM sleep by about 25%. The recommended dosage is 50–150 mg, 30–45 minutes before retiring. Begin with the lower dose for at least three days before increasing it, if necessary.

L-Theanine: Considered helpful for anxiety as well as insomnia. Early research shows that taking 200 mg of theanine (by mouth twice daily for 6 weeks) increases restful sleep and decreases nightly activity during sleep in boys ages 8-12 diagnosed with ADHD.

Melatonin is a hormone produced by the pineal gland in the brain, whose main job is to regulate night and day cycles. Darkness causes the body to produce more melatonin, which signals the body to prepare for sleep. Light decreases melatonin production and signals the body to prepare for being awake. Some people who are sleep-challenged have low levels of melatonin (the amount of which decreases with age), and it may help to add it in supplement form. Success is mixed. Some find it helps, while others feel nothing or else experience vivid dreaming. Standard doses vary: from 500 micrograms all the way up to 10 or 15 milligrams.

Acupoint Break-In: Spleen 9 (Yin Ling Quan, or Yin Mound Spring) is used primarily for digestive issues. It often feels achy or painful with even light stimulus, in great part because most of us have a poor diet. Daily massage helps diminish abdominal pain, distention, diarrhea, edema, urinary incontinence, dysmenorrhea and knee pain. SP9 is on the lower border of the tibia, as shown in the image (SP6 is another important point which we haven't yet discussed). When palpating for the point, always check about an inch below it along the bone and focus on the most tender spot.

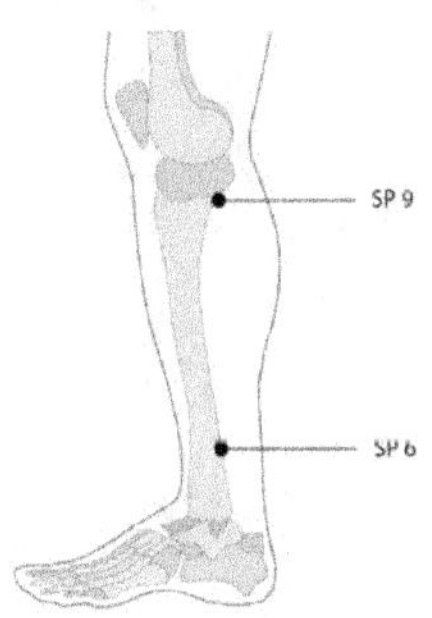

Food for Thought: Acknowledge the Voice.

Equally important as what we ingest is what we allow into our brain. This is especially true for inner voices perhaps that of a parent or boss, that may disrupt your sleep at night. Trying to silence the voice often makes it louder, more insistent. What to do? Make peace with the voice; speak with it. Gently tamp down expectations around sleep. In a hostage situation, you want to negotiate. Be clear.

Thank you for your past service, but I don't need you right now. Speak with the voice as you would with a good friend, or a child struggling to sleep. Use words along these lines: *Remember, there's nothing you have to do, including sleep. Sleep really is no big deal.* Reinforce the sentiment: *It would nice to go to sleep right now, but if I don't, I'll be fine. I'll get some rest, even relax. That's plenty for now. Rest.*

If someone you cared for was struggling with sleep, what would you tell them?

Chapter 11:

Ear-Shaped Box: Auriculotherapy

Your Inner Toolkit

This chapter is built on two premises:

1) The human body has an arsenal of tools for self-repair.

2) We can use heat, as well as pressure, to stimulate acupoints.

Your body is highly resilient, with toolkits for self-repair on the hand, the foot, and on the abdomen among other places. Our focus is on the ear. We can treat anyplace on the body by stimulating an area on the external ear.

Why focus on the ear and not, say, the foot? For one thing, auriculotherapy, as it's called, provides a gateway to the hormonal system. Also, it's a unique subcategory of Chinese medicine, sharing with acupuncture a similar bodily response to stimulation without being bogged down by its complex theory.

Historically, the earliest written records for this therapy appear in China, around 500 BC. Flash forward to 1957 when Dr. Paul Nogier, a French neurologist, introduced auriculotherapy to the West, adding many points that relate to hormonal relationships in the body. In 1991, the U.S. National Institute of Health (NIH) supported auriculotherapy for the relief of pain and for treatment of addiction.

The diagram below shows how we may transpose the body onto the ear. Once you familiarize yourself with the diagram, you can treat other issues as they arise.

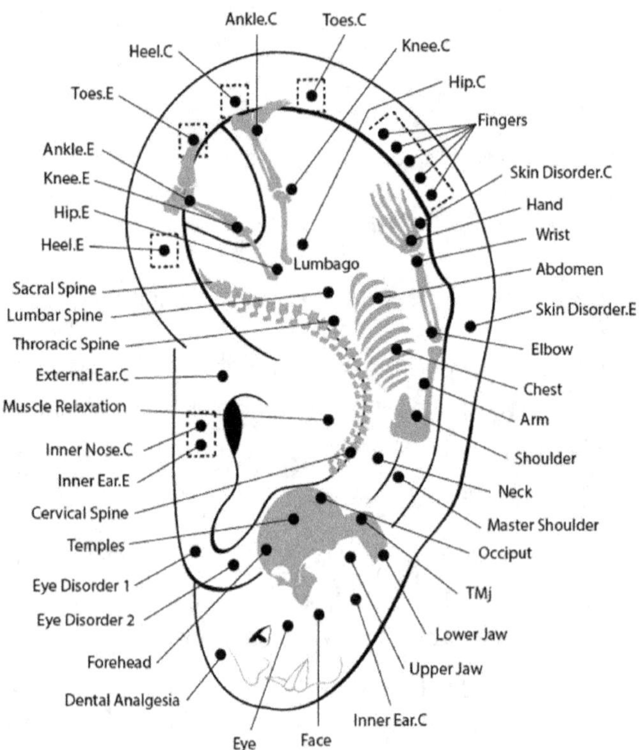

Code:

Round dot = The point is on the surface of the ear.

Square = The point is on the inside flap of the area.

Auriculotherapy Tools:

Q-tip, Tweezer, Ear seeds (small metal balls attached to tape).

Begin by gently massaging your ears for thirty seconds to increase circulation to the area.

1. Use a Q-tip to apply medium pressure to the point.

2. Place ear seeds as shown and massage them often. Leave them in place for three to five days.

3. You'll also be able to use a Tiger Warmer on the points.

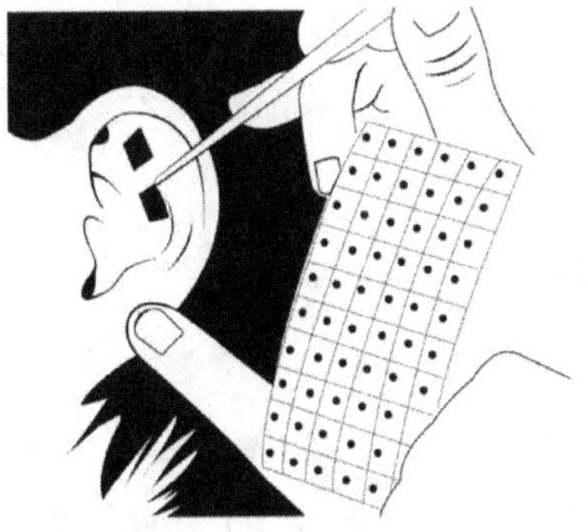

Question: Will the treatment work if I can't reach all the points as shown on your diagram?

Answer: Yes. Our body recalibrates with each point for the best possible outcome.

This is the auricular protocol for insomnia, along with an explanation of the points I used.

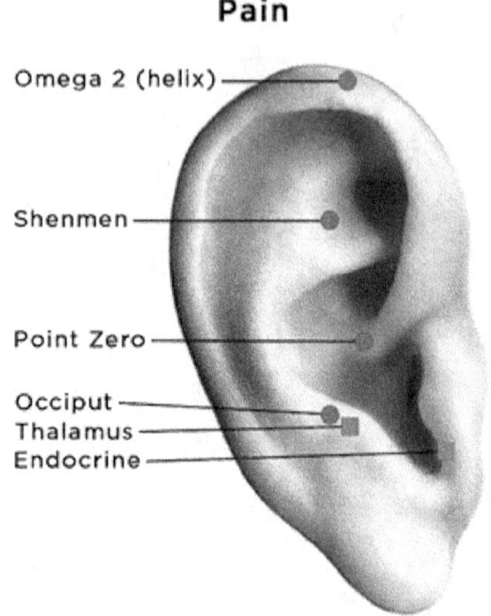

The function of each point is as follows (* indicates higher importance):

*Shenmen: Spirit Gate. Used with almost all auricular treatments, it alleviates pain and anxiety, depression, insomnia, and stressful states.

*Pineal Gland: Helps regulate levels of melatonin, a hormone that regulates sleep function.

Master Cerebral: Lowers chronic pain. It's also where the reflex zones for the prefrontal cortex, or decision-making, are located.

Subcortex — regulates imbalances in brain chemistry.

*Insomnia 1 and 2: Relaxes the body in preparation for sleep. Nervousness, depression.

Brain: Regulates excitation or inhibition of the prefrontal cortex. Affects Pituitary Control. Used for nervous system, digestive, and endocrine dysfunctions. Helps sleep issues.

Tiger Warmers, Heat Therapy

I have already mentioned Tiger Warmers. What are they? There is a tradition in Chinese medicine of using heat as a form of therapy. Classically, a stick made up of a condensed herb (moxa) would be heated and waved over a point. A modern version of this therapy utilizes a guide tube with a spring. It is an effective home tool for heating acupoints. The magic sauce entails thin, incense-like sticks called moxa that are encased in the Tiger Warmer. A spring inside the Warmer makes the heat variable on the skin.

You'll find a tutorial on the use of Tiger Warmers on rewiredforsleep.com.

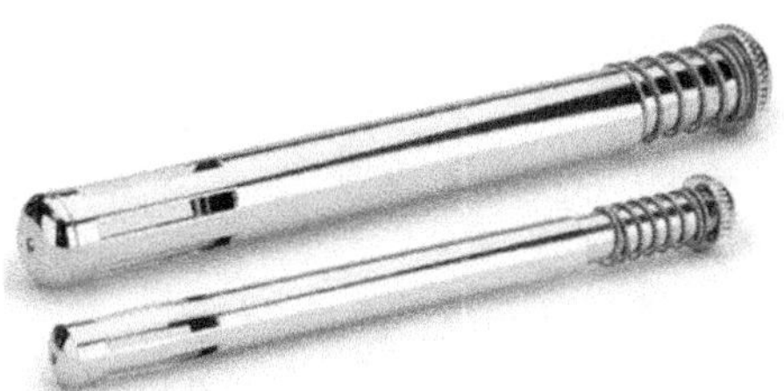

But what is moxa? Moxa is an abbreviation for "moxibustion." It's a spongy herb that, when lighted, is used to heat up an acupoint. The warmth stimulates the flow of Qi and blood to treat gynecological issues, pain, and insomnia among other maladies. This deeply nourishing modality is often a treatment of choice in Asia, where schools are devoted to the study of its proper use. Tiger Warmers are the safest method for the home use of moxa.

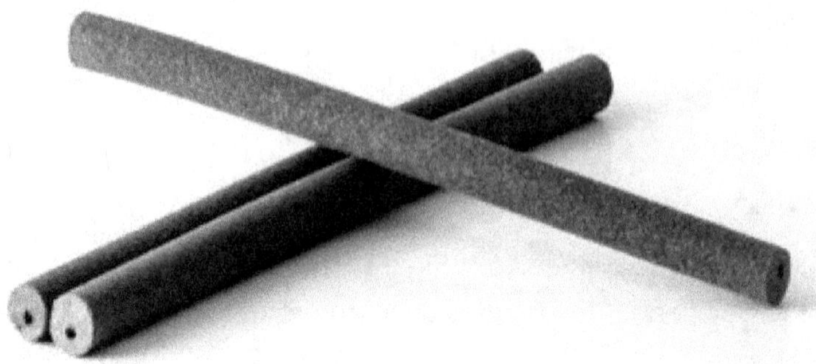

Place a stick of moxa in a Tiger Warmer. There is a spring inside it, so you can move the heat element closer or further from the edge of the metal tube. This lets you control of the heat and provides a calming warmth that penetrates down beneath the skin. You can use a Tiger Warmer on most of the points. After lighting the moxa, touch the Tiger Warmer to the back of your hand before proceeding to make sure the heat is not too great.

The Auricular modules found in the book include: Anxiety, Depression, Digestion, Insomnia, Pain, PTSD, and Stress.

Chapter 12:

The Question of Sleep Aids

Perhaps you believe you need "sleep aids" to get a decent night's rest. That's understandable when you feel you have no other option. The problem? It's a set up. You've been set up to fail in your quest for healthy sleep. This discussion, on what medication does to you, is part one of two; the second section is a primer for quitting the use of any medication in a safe and responsible manner.

"To Dose, Or Not to Dose"

The struggle for sleep invites mind games, second guesses, and even the faux-Bard's query above. Often, the answer is "dose." And that too, is understandable. After you've spent what may feel like a season in sleepless hell, you've tearfully confessed to your doctor that you're at the end of your rope. One hastily scrawled prescription later, and you are good to go. Just then, the slip of paper looks like a ticket out of that hell. Unfortunately, it is all too often a round-trip passage.

Benzodiazepines and the "Z" Drugs: A Primer

The most commonly-used sleep aids are central nervous system depressants. They are also used as anti-anxiety medications, muscle relaxants, antidepressants, and anti-migraines medication. In practice, anti-anxiety and insomnia aids are often used interchangeably.

There are three varying forms of Benzodiazepine. They are rate of absorption into the bloodstream, rate of distribution throughout the body, and how long the drug will remain there. Rapid absorption is more useful for onset insomnia (difficulty getting to sleep), while those with a slower absorption rate are beneficial for maintenance insomnia, or difficulty staying asleep.

The problems with Benzodiazepines are 1) Your body can develop a tolerance to them. 2) When you stop taking them, your body goes into withdrawal. Worst yet, sleeping becomes more difficult than ever, and the possibility of seizures rises.

The "Z" Drugs

This class of sedative-hypnotic drugs includes zolpidem (Ambien), Sonata, and Lunesta. While they have fewer side effects than Benzodiazepines, they are still highly addictive and include barbiturates, antidepressants, and over-the-counter drugs such as antihistamines. They too are habit forming, making sleep even more difficult when a person stops taking them. The laundry list of side-effects for all of these drugs is appalling, and in a sane world would be more than enough reason to ban sleep aids from our shelves forever. They include (this just for Lunesta, chosen here at random):

Day-time drowsiness,

Dizziness,

"Hangover" feeling,

Problems with memory or concentration,

Depression,

Nervous feeling,

Headache

Nausea or vomiting.

Stomach cramps.

Nervousness, anxiety, irritability, or mood swings.

Shakiness or tremors.

Flushing.

Rebound insomnia.

The Facts About Medication

Between 5% and 12% of the adult population now treats insomnia with prescription drugs.

2014 (the last time such statistics were available) saw 60 million prescriptions for sleeping pills, a 30% rise over 2011. The number today is far higher than that.

In 2013, the FDA recommended that women and the elderly use a lower dose of sleep aids. However, only five percent of women and ten percent of the elderly were dispensed lower doses.

> *Show Me the Money*
>
> *According to the American Academy of Sleep Medicine, insomnia in the workplace, and its subsequent absenteeism, costs an annual 63 billion dollars in lost productivity. Add to that all of the associated components, and the numbers are far higher.*

Sleep-aids: What Exactly Do They Do?

We know that the goal of sleep aids is to knock people unconscious; in fact that is their stated function. But don't we want to know if they are restorative? Will taking medication for sleep help you heal, or might taking it mask the underlying problem, thereby making you worse off in the long run? After all, illness does not remain static just because we're not feeling its effects. Before we can answer this question, let's examine the levels or "stages" of sleep we go through on a nightly basis.

The Stages of Sleep

The brain goes through various patterns of activity during sleep. The cycle is a predictable one, and includes two distinct parts — NREM, or Non-REM sleep, plus a REM or "Rapid Eye Movement" cycle. This is what happens in your body during each phase of sleep:

Stage One: Drifting Off: Within minutes (often within seconds) of nodding off, your brain produces what are called alpha and theta waves and your eye movements slow. This introduction to sleep is relatively brief, lasting up to seven minutes. Here, you are in light stage sleep. This means you're somewhat alert and can be easily woken as the brain's beta waves slowly morph into alpha,

and then theta waves. People tend to become most aware of this stage of sleep during catnaps.

Stage Two: Sinking Deeper: The temperature of your body lowers, as does the frequency of your brainwaves. You're moving into deeper relaxation. Stage 2 is home to what are called "sleep spindles"—seemingly random bursts of brainwave activity. Paradoxically, the purpose of these energetic bursts may be to inhibit brain activity to keep you asleep so you can move on to stage 3.

Stage Three: Deep Sleep: This is where the brain begins producing slower delta waves. You won't experience any eye movement or muscle activity. At this point, it gets a little harder for you to be awakened, as your body becomes less responsive to outside stimuli and you move into an even deeper, more restorative stage of sleep. This is when the body repairs muscles and tissues, stimulates growth, boosts immune function, and builds energy for the next day.

Stage Four: REM Sleep: It's during the fourth stage that waking becomes difficult. Most dreaming occurs during this time; your eyes jerk quickly in different directions (hence the name), and heart rate increases. The REM stage is when your brain consolidates and processes information from the previous day, so it can be stored in your long-term memory. This stage is where our brains become active again. Given all that, let's ask, yet again:

Are Sleep Aids Restorative?

Research proved inconclusive, so I decided to ask MDs who specialized in sleep. They would know.

"You tell me" was the near universal reply.

This much we do know: sleep aids increase the amount of medium-depth, non-REM sleep. If you're keeping score, that's non-restorative sleep. The medication doesn't cure you. And the old trope is generally correct: What doesn't make you better will make you sicker. Sadly, someone has dropped the ball when it comes helping those who are sleep deprived.

Of the 90,000 adult emergency room visits annually associated with psychiatric medications, Ambien ranked first, with an estimated 10,212 visits. Ambien is recommended for short-term use only, yet 68% of zolpidem patients were sustained users, with a mean supply of 229 days.

Who is to Blame for Our "Sleep Aid" Problem?

It's not my goal to skewer the medical community. I've worked with physicians whose commitment to helping others was inspiring. They've got trauma down. Life-threatening illness? They're amazing. But when it comes to treating the illnesses with which most people struggle — insomnia, pain, anxiety, digestive issues, and stress — they've been left to wield a single tool: the prescription pad. The medical community has tossed in the white towel and rolled over for the pharmaceutical industry. To paraphrase the old hammer and nail metaphor, when all you have is a prescription pad, everyone needs a pill.

Big Pharma likes this worldview. It would cost hundreds of millions of dollars to vet new methods; Return on Investment would be negligible. For a business model based on repeat customers, as that one is, the phrase "long-term cure" is as inviting to shareholders as garlic is to a vampire. We needn't be surprised that new treatment methods remain untested.

What's more, even if your MD has been exposed to the therapies outlined here, she can't be properly compensated for the time needed to dispense them. There's no medical code for "teach abdominal breathing" or any of the tools available here. No code, no money, no treatment.

The use of psychoactive drugs isn't just a modern phenomenon. The Aztecs were known to use herbs to treat anxiety and depression. But would you be surprised to hear that their skills in psychopharmacology weren't all benign?

Aztec priests considered anxiety to be a bad omen for prisoners awaiting sacrifice. With their access to psychoactive herbs like peyote and psilocybin mushroom they gave condemned prisoners a brew so they wouldn't despair and thereby offend the gods.

So, a blood-smeared priest is about to carve out my heart, slather molé sauce on it and then eat it before a screaming throng? I'll pass.

Let's set aside Aztec Prozac and Veracruz Valium, and instead use gentle acupressure to deflate anxiety. Two commonly used points are Heart 7 and Pericardium 6.

Heart 7: Spirit Gate

Heart 7 (HT7, Shenmen, or Spirit Gate), is an acupoint used to reduce insomnia, disturbing dreams, and palpitations. In Chinese medicine, each organ has both a physiological function and an emotional one. Let's remember that Western medicine tells us that the stomach has its own "brain." And don't we all know someone with a "nervous stomach"? In keeping with that idea, the heart does more than pump blood. It's also involved with sleep and sleep-related emotions. HT7 is located on the pinky side of the wrist crease, on the inside of the ligament that attaches the hand to the arm.

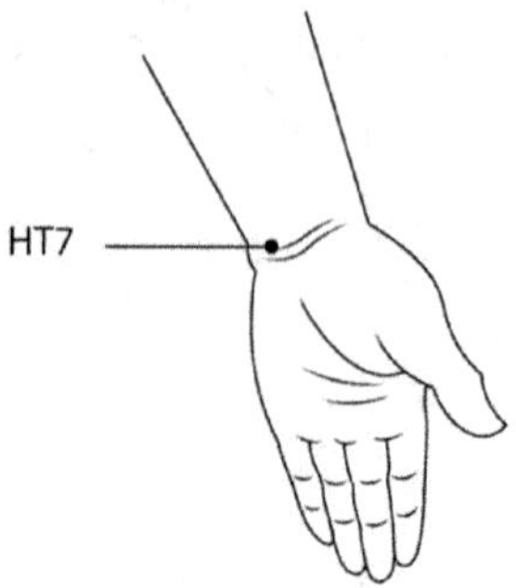

Pericardium 6: Inner Pass

A point that is related to HT7 is Pericardium 6 (PC6, Neiguan; Inner Pass). The physiological role of the pericardium is that of heart protector. PC6 serves that function by relieving anxiety, palpitations, insomnia, nausea, and irritability. Wristbands that stimulate PC6 are available to women who are pregnant and experiencing nausea, or for those who experience sea-sickness (again, here is the brain-stomach connection). Locate the point three finger widths up from the wrist crease, between the two major tendons.

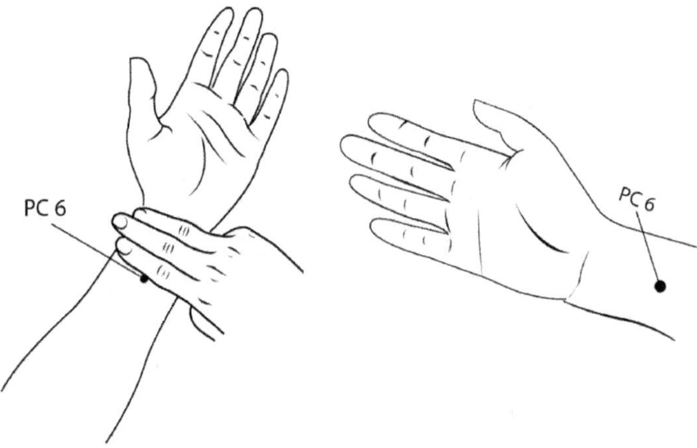

If you're experiencing anxiety, put aside five minutes to massage these points twenty-four times in each direction. Soon, we'll bring other therapies into play and incorporate these points into them.

Chapter 13:

In Her Mind, She Left it All Behind

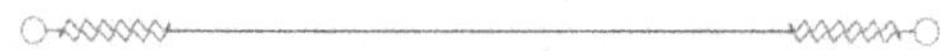

Dina Hangs Her Problems on a Hook

With her upswept hair displaying a high forehead atop round, acid green eyeglasses, and alabaster skin that bears no trace of having encountered makeup, there is a no-nonsense aspect to Dina.. She sits across from me scanning my diplomas, my Meridian Man, the auricular poster.

"I've always been a ... happy person," she begins. "No issues, or none to speak of. I always slept like a baby. That's changed in the last year. I'm thinking of tossing it all — the job, the home, even the boyfriend — and heading for Hawaii. It's stress."

"I understand. Anything in particular spark it off?"

She shakes her head.

"I knew it was bad when I was waking up at five a.m. For no reason! On weekends. I do yoga." She clenches her jaw. "What else can I do?"

"Leave it all behind."

Her jaw drops. I quickly explain myself, lest she think I'm serious. So what if Hawaii is sounding pretty good on a gray and chilly November day, in New York town?

"It's easy to say, leave the workday behind before coming home, but given the demands of life, hard to do. You take work-related calls as you're walking in the front door, right?"

"Of course. What else am I supposed to do?"

"Start unwinding your nervous system twenty minutes before getting home. That's when you end work-related calls and put away the phone. There are times when I walk around the block before entering my home. Sometimes I do it twice. And no, that's not a time to get back on the phone.

 "I've got a friend who's a social worker," I say. "She visits people who have been abused, people who feel lost or hopeless, people who are ill and feel all alone. The things she deals with on a daily basis would make a grown man cry. We worked at the same clinic and became friends. One night, we were about to grab a bite when we stopped by her place to pick up something. As we got inside, she took off her coat, did some wavy movements with her hands, gazed into the mirror, made a few faces, and then continued about her business as if nothing had happened.

"She then went in and hugged her little daughter like any happy solo mom would do. I was curious about the miming in the hallway and asked what it was about. She told me that after having her daughter, she'd knew she'd need to protect her from the negative energy. So when she walks in the door now, she takes off her work face, hangs the day's problems on a hook, and locates in the mirror the joyful smile she's been saving up for her daughter.

"She doesn't have to worry about the world's problems for another twelve hours. They're there by the door, hanging out, while she goes about her life. Next morning, she picks them up again on the way out, by which time, some are gone, and the others have shrunk."

Dina listens intently. On her way out she turns and says, half to herself,

"Maybe heaven can wait awhile."

Dina Creates a Model for Tranquility

Before leaving work, Dina imagines a dustbin by her desk and mentally dumps the day's accumulated junk in it. When she is home, she takes off her "office self" and hangs it up for the evening. Before leaving for work in the morning, she puts on her "office self" and heads out. At night, before getting in bed, Dina goes through her checklist.

A week before the arrival of her period she typically gets PMS with pain, bloating, moodiness, and tender breasts. Two acupoints in particular can help relieve symptoms: Liver 3 and Spleen 6 (SP6, Sanyinjiao, or Three Yin Connection). A crossroads point for meridians impacting on the mind, SP6 sits four finger-widths above the tip of the inner anklebone. Press along the bone and find the achy spot for abdominal or back pain, bloating, diarrhea, edema, hernia, headache, and dizziness

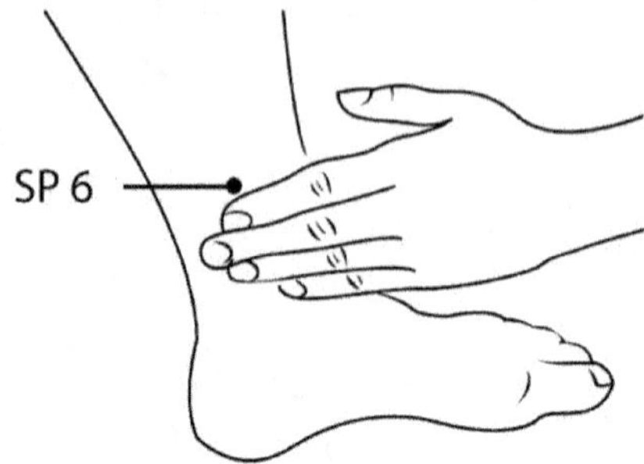

The other point is Liver 3 (LV3, Tai Chong, Great Rushing). Since the liver is the organ of Detoxification (both physical and, in the view of Chinese medicine, emotional), it makes sense that stress-related toxins go to the liver. A toxic liver creates heat, which, in that world view, rises up to disturb the mind to create insomnia. LV3 not only helps with sleep, it eases anger and frustration, PMS, and lumbar pain. Not so coincidentally, it calms digestive issues including nausea, vomiting, or diarrhea, and helps ease itchy, red eyes as well. Find Liver 3 on the top of the foot in a small depression between the first and second toes (see illustration)

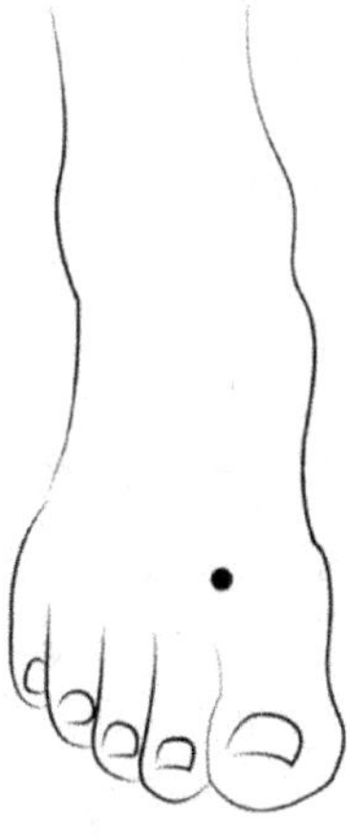

Liver 3

In our stressed-out culture, LV3 is often sensitive to pressure. Take a few minutes in the evening to massage it, or use a Tiger Warmer while you're watching TV or reading.

When Dina feels overwhelmed, she "checks in" for five minutes of self-care. Her go-to method is the Butterfly Hug.

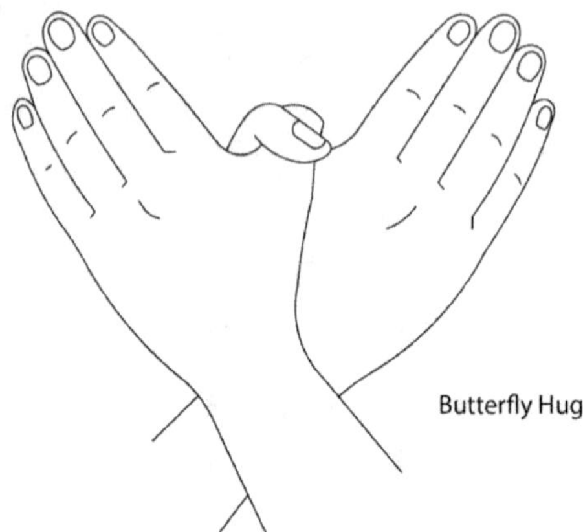

Butterfly Hug

Exercise 11: The Butterfly Hug

This antidote to stress and trauma was created by Lucina Artigas, during her work with survivors of Hurricane Pauline in Acapulco, Mexico in 1998. Despite its almost absurd simplicity, Butterfly Hug is a highly effective treatment, utilizing both bilateral stimulation and a powerful acupoint called Kidney 27.

Cross your arms over your chest, so the tip of the middle finger from each hand sits below the collarbone. The other fingers rest naturally under the collarbone. Hands and fingers must be as vertical as possible, so that the fingers point toward the neck and not toward the arm. Your index fingers should touch what we know as the collarbone point in Meridian Tapping, and which in Chinese medicine is called Kidney 27, shown here:

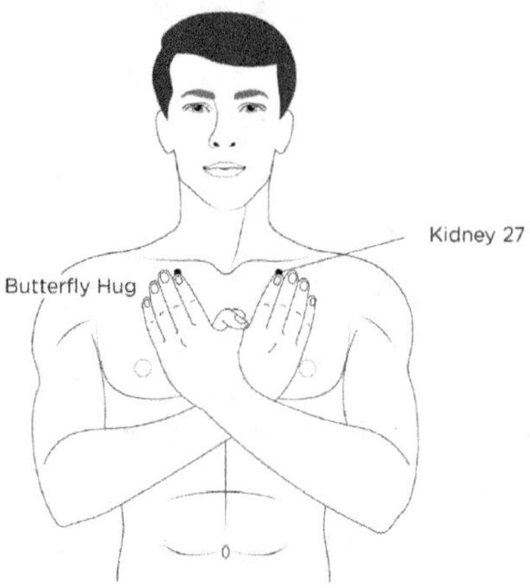

Interlock your thumbs to form the butterfly's body. The extension of your other fingers forms the Butterfly's wings. Your eyes can be closed, or partially closed. As you alternate the movement of your hands, like the flapping wings of a butterfly, notice any thoughts, images, sounds, and sensations going through you. If you feel stressed, close your eyes, take three deep breaths, and use the Butterfly Hug.

Dina learns the Staircase. In this guided visualization she descends a set of stairs, at the bottom of which is a door that opens to a special place.

Exercise 12: Staircase to Your Special Place (V-K)

Listen to the guided meditation for The Staircase at https://rewiredforsleep.com/guided-meditations.

The Staircase

Take a deep breath in, hold it, and as you let it out, let your eyes relax. Take another deep breath in, and as you exhale, close your eyes.

In a moment, you'll descend a staircase, and as you do so, you'll start counting from ten down to one. For the first five steps, imagine you're opening your eyes and then closing them. As you inhale, open them, and close them on the exhale. Breathe gently. It's easy once you get into the rhythm of it: inhale and imagine you're opening your eyes, exhale and close.

See yourself at the top of a set of stairs. They might be made of wood, or stone, or metal, or some other material. There might be a handrail, and it might be ornate or simple. There are ten steps, and you're standing at the top, looking down. Inhale, and as you land on a step, exhale and imagine a wave of relaxation rolling down your body. Inhale and take another step down.

Staircase

Starting at Ten, eyes open, inhale. As you go down to step

Nine, exhale and close your eyes, and feel that wave of relaxation.

Open eyes and another breath in. As you go down to

Eight, close your eyes and exhale. Feel another wave of relaxation.

Open your eyes, and breathe in. As you go down to

Seven, breathe out and close your eyes. See the wave of relaxation.

Six. Eyes open, breathe in, and on the out breath, close your eyes, down to

Five. More relaxed now, and with your next three, relaxing breaths, experience a wave of relaxation from the top of your head, down to the tips of your toes, and beyond. Down to

Four. Breathing comfortably now, deeply relaxed, down to

Three. Breathing in, and out. And inhale. Stepping down to

Two, and breathe out. As you get to

One. At the bottom of stairs, you'll see a door before you. Notice the color of the door. Notice whether it pulls in or pushes out. Open the door and enter your special place. Dina pulls open a door and goes out to her Special Place, which for her is a seaside villa on Oahu.

Dina sees herself in a boat, drifting out, past city lights and under a star-filled night sky, through dark rivers out to a fathomless sea. The gentle rocking of the boat lulls her sleep.

Chapter 14:

Herbal Options

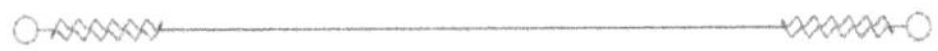

Sleep-Positive Herbs

We've used herbs for their sedative properties ever since one Cro Mag lost sleep coveting his neighbor's cave, or wife, or both. The advent of powerful drugs nearly sounded the death knell for medicinal herbs in the West until recently, amid renewed interest in treating health issues with natural methods. It seems the pendulum has begun to swing back in their favor, and with good reason. Herbs tend to work subtly, have relatively few side effects and, unlike sleep drugs, are non-addictive.

Chinese herbal formulas are also entering into the mainstream of awareness. The product of centuries of meticulous tinkering, most prescriptions are constructed to target specific symptoms using multiple herbs, even as they mitigate potential side effects. 3000 year-old Chinese herbology is an elegant, fully realized system unto itself, with a depth and beauty that's still unparalleled in the West.

Can't get to sleep and tend to run cold? Your prescription would differ from that of someone who wakes at 2 a.m., kicking off their covers because they're overheated. Given all the variables involving sleep issues, it's best to see a licensed herbal practitioner of Chinese herbs whenever possible.

Western Herbs

Western herbs tell a different story. Unlike formulas, they rarely address underlying problems, but they tend to be fast-acting. The following herbs are often used for sleep issues:

Hops (Humulus lupulus):

Hops as a reputation for being a sedative specifically for insomnia due to worry or jangled nerves. Dose: Tea, 1 cup 2-3 x daily; Tincture, 30-40 drops 2-3 x daily.

Valerian (Valeriana officinalis) :

Six percent of Americans use Valerian for insomnia, nervousness, and restlessness. Used mainly by those who are having a hard time falling asleep, it's said to also reduce night-time waking. May be used in combination with California poppy, skullcap, hops, and passion flower. Dose: Tea, 1 cup; Tincture, 2-5 droppers-full 2-3 x daily.

Kava (Piper methysticum):

Native to the western Pacific region, indigenous cultures have used Kava for over three thousand years. It's often used to treat sleeplessness, anxiety, depression, and fatigue. Not recommended if you are taking antiplatelet medications; anticoagulants (Coumadin) or antipsychotic medications. Dose: Tea, 1 cup; Tincture, 3-4 droppers full 2-3 x daily.

Chamomile:

Safe for children and adults alike. In tea form, it's often used for insomnia, restlessness, and irritability. Chamomile oil can be put in bath water (5-6 drops) to soothe nerves, diluted to two percent to make an excellent massage oil, or used as an inhalant (S).

Dose: Tea, 1 cup 2-3 x daily; Tincture, 30 drops 3 x daily.

Combination: chamomile and oat straw tea for insomnia and anxiety (courtesy of Anna Almiroudis)

Passionflower (Passiflora):

Passionflower has been used for hundreds of years for its ability to reduce anxiety, or stress-related insomnia. Excellent for people experiencing emotional volatility.

CBD (Cannabidiol):

The latest kid on the healing block, Cannabidiol is said to treat everything from neurological disorders to chronic pain and depression. Some of its fans claim it reduces anxiety and helps them sleep; others report that it has a caffeine-like effect on them. Dosages vary despite what may be indicated. Among the sleep disorders for which CBD has shown to provide relief are Circadian Rhythm disorders, which often affects people with night-time jobs.

St. John's Wort (Hypericum perforate):

A commonly found European herb, many people use St. John's Wort to alleviate mild depression, as well as for treating chronic insomnia. The herb may increase your skin's sensitivity to the sun. If you take this herb, try not to expose your skin to direct sunlight. Dose: Tincture, 1/2 to 1 teaspoon 2-3 x daily; powdered extract, 1-2 tablets or capsules 2-3 x daily. Allow 2-3 weeks for the full therapeutic effect to develop.

California Poppy :

Can provide mental calmness, decrease anxiety, and ease restless feelings. Often used as a tincture, you take 30-40 drops of it before bed each night.

Cordyceps Sinensis:

Cordyceps helps those suffering with stress-induced adrenal fatigue, which is often tied in with insomnia. Traditional healers recommend the fungus/mushroom as a general tonic to improve energy, appetite, and endurance, and to stabilize sleeping patterns.

Western Herbal Formulas for Insomnia

Even with Western herbs, it's safer to use a formula over an individual herb, and these two blends are effective. If you're unfamiliar with some of the herbs in them, they've been included for their safety.

A CALMING TEA BLEND:

Linden flowers (1 part)

Hawthorn flowers & leaves (1 part)

Chamomile (2 parts)

Catnip (1 part)

Lemon balm (1 part)

Wintergreen (1 part),

Stevia herb (1/8 part)

BEDTIME TEA:

Valerian (30%)

Linden (20%)

Kava kava (20%)

Chamomile (20%)

Catnip (10%)

Blend the loose herbs, then place in a quart jar for future use, and store out of the direct sunlight in a cool place. Use 1 tsp/cup to make a tea. Make 1 quart at a time, adding 1 extra tsp "for the pot." Add the herbs to boiled water and cover. Let steep for 20 minutes, strain, and store in the quart jar in the refrigerator. This blend will keep for 3 days. Pour out 1 cup, warm it, and drink several times daily or before bedtime as needed. As usual, they may take some time to take effect, so patience is required.

Herbal Break-In: Turmeri-Cola!

A member of the ginger family and a mainstay in Ayurvedic medicine, turmeric grows mainly in India and Indonesia. The herb can reduce pain, inflammation, and stiffness related to rheumatoid arthritis and osteoarthritis. It treats bursitis, is a natural liver detoxifier, and is a kidney cleanser. Besides aiding metabolism in weight loss, turmeric can alleviate depression, psoriasis, and damaged skin. It helps almost all things sleep-related, without putting you to sleep. Why include it? When you're healthy, you tend to sleep better. It's that simple.

For Turmeric-Cola you will need:

10-12 pieces of turmeric

5-7 tamarind fruit

2-3 lemons

raw honey

water

blender

strainer

bowl

glass jar with lid

1. Peel turmeric. Your fingers will turn yellow, but fret not. All-natural dish soap gets it out. (Scrub! Or use rubber gloves.) If your cutting board gets stained, use dish soap. Let it soak in for five minutes or so, then scrub with water and sponge. Crack and open the tamarind. Make sure you get all the roots off, too. We'll use only the fruit.

2. Fill a pot with water, toss peeled turmeric in and let it boil for twenty to thirty minutes, or until the water turns a vibrant marigold color.

3. While it's boiling, get a pan and pour 1 inch of water in, adding the peeled tamarind. Move the fruit around with a wooden spoon, mixing it with the water so the tamarind dissolves into a jam-like texture. Add water as needed. By this time, you should see the little seeds. When the texture is soft, turn the heat off the pan, and let it cool down.

4. Pour just enough cold water into the turmeric water to lower the temperature. Pour the mixture into the blender with the softened turmeric pulp for flavor. Before blending, make sure it's cooled, otherwise the heat can create too

much pressure in a blender. (Let's say I now know better ways to kill an hour than to spend it wiping turmeric juice off kitchen walls.) Blend. The color will now be a fiery marigold.

5. Pour the tamarind into a strainer over a bowl to catch what's left. Swish it around in the strainer with the wooden spoon — we only want the soft stuff, no seeds.

6. Place the jam-like stuff into the blender with the turmeric water. If it's gloppy, pick out the seeds and roots and place the rest into the blender. Blend again.

7. Squeeze the lemons and add the juice in the blender. Zap. Pour your juice into the jar. Add honey to taste, close the lid, shake it up to mix.

Store in your refrigerator for up to 3-4 days and partake to your heart's content.

Chapter 15:

Unplug from Anxiety

Anxiety, Sleep Killer #1

Insomnia that's based in anxiety tends to arise either in the prefrontal cortex or in the amygdala. If you typically talk yourself into a state of anxiety, it starts at the prefrontal cortex; if you're jolted into anxiety, then it's probably amygdala based. We'll see how either kind can disrupt sleep.

Edward, 31, is a single dad struggling with insomnia and amygdala-based panic attacks. He sports a gray track suit, and black visor cap turned backward over wispy blond hair.

"Used to be I'd wake up at two a.m. for half-hour," he says, "then fall asleep again. Now, I'm awake till five, but then it's almost time to get up for work. The panic's worst part of it."

"How does it manifest?"

"Palpitations. Sweating. Mind racing. Crazy thoughts."

His parents divorced when he was nine. At age twelve, he woke one night to strange sounds coming from his older sister's room. Alarmed, he peeked in and saw her being sexually abused by their mother's boyfriend. The sight of his sister in a helpless state devastated the young boy, but he said nothing. For years after, Edward suffered with depression and panic attacks. Insomnia was a recent and unwanted added burden. He shares with me that he is terrified that he is losing his mind.

"Panic can happen anywhere. I might be in a restaurant with my daughter laughing, and suddenly, for no reason, my hands sweat, my heart races and I'm crazy out of control."

Anxiety thrives when the left and right sides of the brain are not communicating. To get both sides of the brain talking to one another, we can use a form of bilateral stimulation called "Four-Step Trauma Intervention." This simple exercise that can go far toward settling an anxious mind.

Exercise 13: Four-Step Trauma Intervention (FSTI)

As described by Jeannette Amlie, Four-Step Trauma Intervention has four sections: Notice, Interrupt, Discharge, and Re-Pattern.

"Next time that you feel a sense of dread or panic," I tell Edward, "acknowledge its presence. Say to yourself, I feel overwhelmed right now. That alone changes how your brain processes it. Next, we use left-right stimulation by going across your body from your dominant side to the other side to interrupt the pattern. You left or right-handed?"

"Righty." Clearly in no mood for games, Edward is desperate enough to try anything. Even this.

"Bilateral stimulation's as easy as tapping your left knee with your right hand."

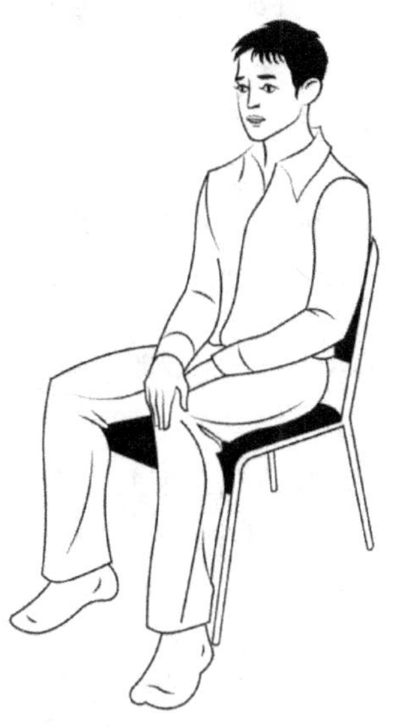

"I could do that."

"You can also toss a ball, an apple or any object between your hands."

"Could I scratch my right cheek with my left hand?"

"Yes! That's the 'Interrupt.' Next you 'Discharge': yawn, shake, sigh. Then shake out your body to release the trauma. from muscle memory while re-booting your nervous system. That's Re-pattern."

I prescribe a formula containing ginseng, astragalus, atractylodis and honey baked licorice root to boost his energy and ease the palpitations. I also suggest that he enlist a talk therapist.

"It's a bigger commit than I'm capable of right now," he says. "Can we do hypnosis in the meantime?" Since trance work is often used as a bridge to therapy, I agree to work with him.

Once Edward is in trance, I ask him if he is ready to explore the deeper levels of his mind. Only after he nods "yes," do I guide him forward. On his own, Edward uncovers that he has been punishing himself for not saving his sister that night for fear of harming his tenuous relationship with their mother. His sadness in describing the terrible roots of his insomnia is very real just then.

"Are you ready to let go of punishing yourself?" I ask, in a neutral manner. I know it's a big ask, and I would not be surprised if he answered with a resounding "no". Minutes tick by in silence. It's very possible that he isn't about to let himself off the hook.

"I'm done," he replies with greater force than I had expected.

I have him recall a time in his life when he felt strong and confident. I then "anchor" the memory with a post-hypnotic suggestion that he'll use positive experiences to replace negative ones as they arise. I slowly emerge him.

At night, if Edward has a panic attack. he uses the Butterfly Hug, then mentally descends a staircase to his "Special Place". For him, it is a lakeside cabin. [Find the Lake in the Extra Mile 1.5]

Update: Edward is sleeping more profoundly, and with fewer interruptions, than at any time since he was twelve. He goes to a woman therapist with whom he feels safe, even as he continues to receive acupuncture. As the fog of depression slowly lifts, he is starting to locate inner peace at long last.

Jenna Reclaims Her Brain (Prefrontal Cortex Anxiety)

Jenna, 55, is a high school art teacher in Babylon, Long Island. Wavy strawberry blond hair frames her broad face, and flower tattoos stream down arms kissed by a lifetime of sun worship. She has difficulty getting to sleep due to anxiety, which she describes as "a slow-moving squall roiling my insides". She also has knee pain, a residue of her younger, wilder, rugby-playing days.

> "Before I'm even in bed, my brain's talking to me. 'Jenna,' she's saying, 'you're not sleeping tonight. Tomorrow you're going to feel like shit.' The closer I get to bedtime, the meaner 'she' gets. By the time I put my head on the pillow, I'm up for the count. It stinks." From the way Jenna describes her anxiety, we may assume it is rooted in her prefrontal cortex.

Fear of being unable to get to sleep has a name: Psycho-physiological Insomnia.

> "What prompted me to take the Zoloft," she tells me, "is my son Joey. He's hooked on pain pills. We don't talk much these days." She nabs a nearby tissue. "But I so want to help him."

> "Let's try something," I say, "called the Four-Step-Trauma Intervention."

Jenna does Four-Step Trauma Intervention

> "Is there anything in particular that triggers you?" I ask.

> "It's random. I could be at home or teaching a class, when I'll imagine something happening to Joey, always a worst case scenario. It's like a wave that starts at my left temple and slowly rolls through me." She shivers as if for emphasis.

"To diminish the feeling," I reply, "we first want to see how it moves through us. Then we interrupt the pattern. But if you're in front of your class, you need to be subtle to get the right/left, right left activity going. Could you squeeze your butt cheeks, first right, then left in groups of three?"

She nods her head yes, even as she lets out a barely stifled grin.

"The next step is to discharge energy: You might sigh or stretch, or even laugh."

"No problem."

"Finally, you Re-pattern. Do something physical in order to reboot your system. Maybe it means you'll step out to the hall for a minute, stretch, or hum a few bars of your favorite song. Again, it's Notice, Interrupt, Discharge and Re-Pattern." She nods her head and repeats the sequence to me.

I show her two acupoints that help ease anxiety. One is Yintang, and the other one is Pericardium 6.

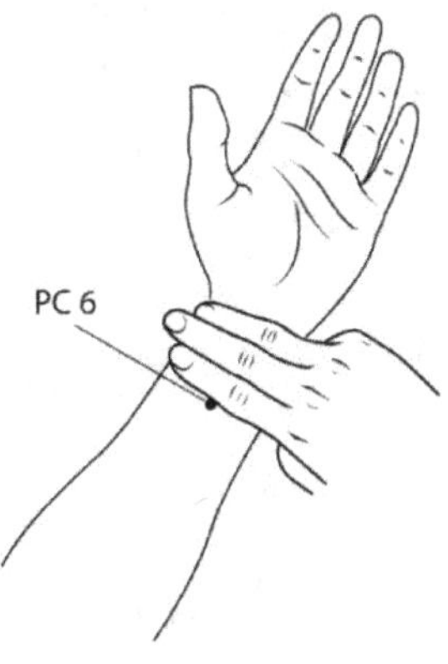

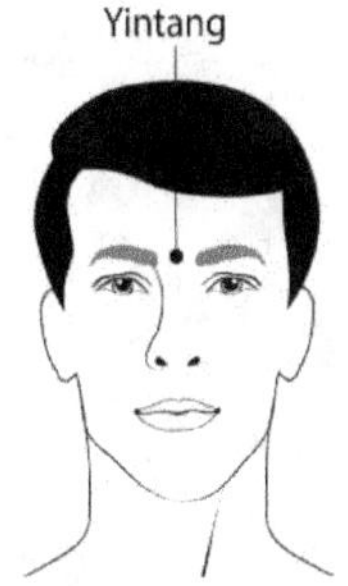

"At night," I say, "begin by taking several deep belly breaths, then gently massage each point twenty-four times."

Jenna takes 5-HTP, an amino acid that the body naturally produces to help make serotonin. She listens to the Autogenic Training recording, and the anxiety eases, little by little.

"If I wake up in a panic — it happens — Autogenic Training or FSTI helps. So does Acknowledge the Voice. Knowing I've got options, is major."

What still can keep her on tenterhooks is anxiety around the wellbeing of her son. I mention ALANON, a 12-Step group for people caught in the wake of substance abusers. She finds a nearby meeting and quickly connects with members. Most of them have been through sagas like Jenna's, and found a well of inner strength that carries them forward. One woman offers to take Jenna under her wing, and Jenna, fiercely independent in most other regards, agrees to accept her help.

Jenna's new friend from ALANON takes her to a meditation meeting. She finds it hard to sit still at first, but then commits to a daily meditation practice. All told, she is now sleeping more deeply and with far fewer fits and starts than she has in many years.

"I've let go," she tells me, "of a lot. And it's all good."

Since Jenna has turned a corner and is sleeping better, we terminate treatment.

Six months later, an email shows up in my inbox. Jenna's sleeping better, if imperfectly. When anxiety rears its head, she can usually nab it before it can kill her night. As an aside, she comments that Joey has found a way to stay clean without the help of his mother. He is studying audio engineering at a local college, and very happy. I thank her for the follow up.

Chapter 16:

Fatigue, and Refilling the Empty Well

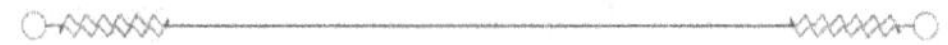

Michelle Hits the Wall

Michelle is happily divorced, with two boys, nine and six. You wouldn't know from her good-natured laugh that she struggles with anxiety and fatigue. At age 42, she finds it harder to get to sleep than to stay asleep and is often exhausted. Fatigue impacts on her social life and on the copywriting job. It is the work fatigue that scares her. With her gray-streaked, Joan Jett-black hair, piercing dark eyes, and angular cheekbones, I could imagine her in the old West, driving a wagon train.

"What's real bad," Michelle tells me, "is that my yoga practice — my go-to support system — is failing me." Puffiness under her eyes is probably due to sleep deficiency and anxiety medication.

> "Sure, there's work stress," Michelle says, "but I love a good laugh. Sex has always been big for me, but these days I feel like my libido's waning. Which sucks. On top of that, I've put on these goddamn fifteen pounds. I think my hormones are way out of whack.

Tests indicate that she is dealing with adrenal fatigue. This little-addressed issue is everywhere in our stressed-out culture; I see children running on empty before they are even out of high school. This contributes to ADHD, to increased levels of obesity, and to depression. So, what are the adrenals, and if they're in fact, fatigued, how do we fix them?

Adrenal Fatigue

Seated atop both the left and right kidneys are two glands called the adrenals. These small, workhorse glands control the secretion of many hormones into our bloodstream. One such hormone, adrenaline, gets us up in the morning, while cortisol is our perennial stress hormone. If you are anxious, or sensitive, or easily overwhelmed, your cortisol levels spike in response to situations that your nervous system perceives as stressful. Each time that happens, the adrenals get a little bit more drained. If you're exhausted but still can't sleep, you might be suffering from adrenal fatigue. Symptoms include:

- Waking up feeling tired no matter how much you have slept.

- Being less able to handle stress than you used to.

- You're still gaining weight despite working out and eating within range of your size.

- You are emotionally volatile for no reason

- You have odd memory lapses

- You experience muscle weakness

- Climbing stairs, which shouldn't be a problem for you, is exhausting

- You feel lightheaded coming out of Downward Dog

Adrenal Repair

Acupressure: KI6 and KI27

Acupoint Kidney 6 (KI6, Zhao Hai, Shining Sea) is often enlisted to treat menopausal conditions such as hot flashes, night sweats, insomnia, and vaginal dryness, along with menstrual disorders. It's also used for such symptoms as palpitations, anxiety, sore throat, and adrenal fatigueLocate KI6 just below the inner ankle bone, called the medial malleolus, as shown in the diagram.

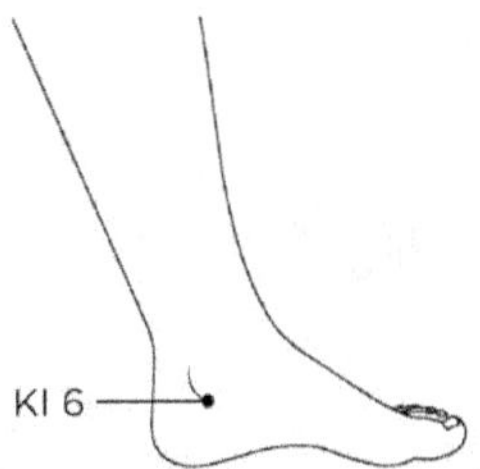

Kidney 27=Collarbone Point

Kidney 27, or Collarbone Point, sits on both sides of the chest. Trace your collarbones toward the center of your chest until your fingers almost meet in the middle. You'll notice two nodes before the collarbone dips to form a "V."

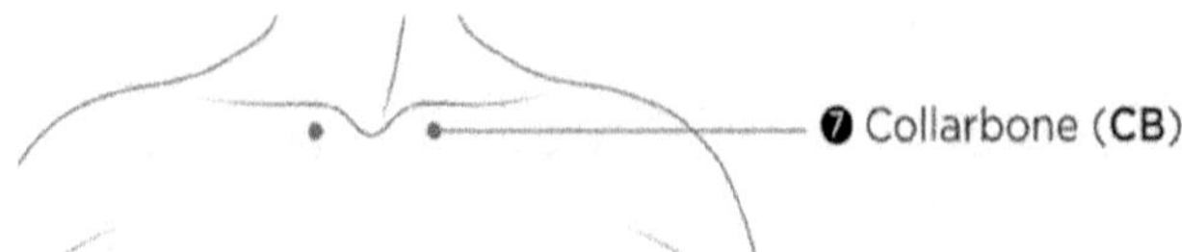

Bring your fingers down and out toward each side of your body about an inch, and you'll find a depression under the collarbones. Press on those two points. If one of them is painful (often the left), you may have adrenal fatigue.

Supplements: Vitamin B, especially B-12. Vitamin C (Solgar or Jarrow brand)

VITAMIN D3—A deficiency of Vitamin D3 can be a cause of difficulty sleeping. Have your Vitamin D levels checked. Low vitamin D is associated with fibromyalgia and with insomnia.

Herb: Cordyceps Sinensis

Essential Oils: Ylang Ylang

"Anxiety's eating me up," Michelle says, "and I will not take drugs just now. What else have you got?"

"This is a job for Reverse Spin."

"Beg your pardon?" A shadow of concern slides across Michelle's normally impassive face.

Exercise 14: The Reverse Spin

You can see a video demonstrating Reverse Spin at rewiredforsleep.com/the-deeper-levels.

The Reverse Spin is a method created by Richard Bandler, one of the originators of Neuro-Linguistic Programming. It's made for people who are in a deeply negative emotional state.

"We tend to think our emotions are in our head, but they're actually in our body as well," I tell her. "The first thing you want to do is to locate where in your body that negative feeling sits."

"I haven't got a clue where it is," says Michelle.

"It might be in your chest, your belly, or your head —take a moment to feel it in your body."

Michelle taps her chest lightly. "It's here," she says in a low voice.

"How would you rate the discomfort on a scale from one to ten, with ten being worst??"

"Seven point five?"

"Here's the other thing: emotions aren't static. They move around inside of us. Basically, it's energy and has a polarity attached to it. And the energy moves. If it didn't, it would dissipate, so it spins, rotating back its starting point and then back again. Notice how it's spinning." I demonstrate how it's done by rotating my left arm before me. "Thing is, it typically moves clockwise or counterclockwise, left or right. Which way do you feel it'll go for you?"

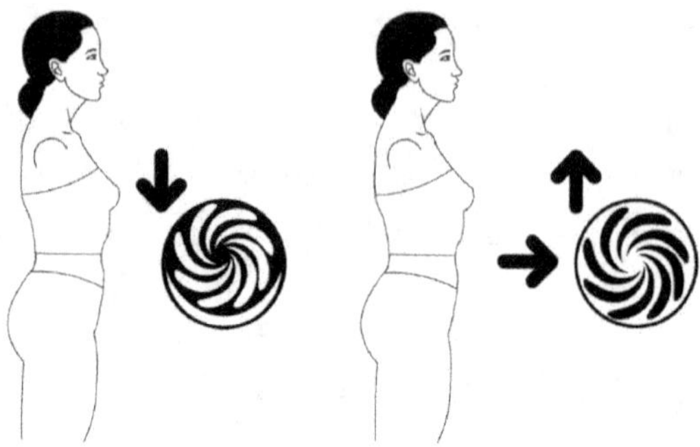

She rotates her hand in a small tight circle, hesitantly at first, in a clockwise motion.

"It's like a wheel before me," she says.

"Now, imagine you can bring that wheel outside and in front of your body."

Michelle continues rotating her arm outside of her body in a widening arc.

"Now reverse the movement," I say, "from clockwise to counterclockwise. Move your arm in the opposite direction and slowly bring it back into your body. At this point you've shifted the energetic polarity. Your body is incapable of processing both directions; they essentially nullify one another."

Michelle moves her hand back to her chest and holds it before her. She stops moving her hand.

"Breathe, hold it for three seconds, and exhale. What number is the discomfort now?"

"I don't know. A two, maybe? This is very strange."

Michelle repeats the exercise. The anxiety appears to have melted away.

"Feels like something's shifted," she says, "I'll grant you that."

She purchases a Tiger Warmer and starts using it on LV3 and on SP6.

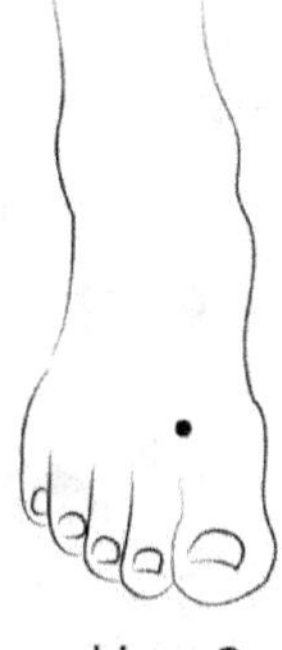

Liver 3

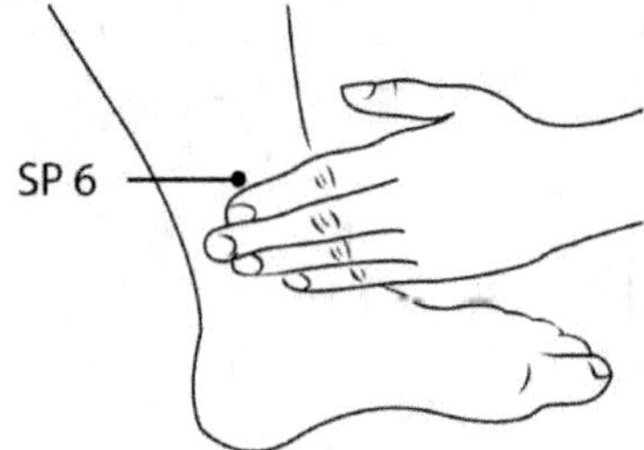

Michelle has been getting treatment twice a week for four weeks. Now that she has regained control of her nervous system, she feels stronger. As a result, we start tapering her visits. Michelle now comes in weekly, then once a month. She is also doing her beloved Ashtanga yoga again.

"I'd kind of given up hope of sleeping," she says. "Now, after twenty minutes I'm usually gone to dreamland. And that's without my two glasses of Merlot. Okay, I'm down to one. And," she says, "my sex drive is back, baby! I hope that's not TMI!" A lusty laugh punctuates this rhetorical question.

Michelle continues to come in for tune-ups, as needed.

Bonus Ear Protocol: Stress

Stress

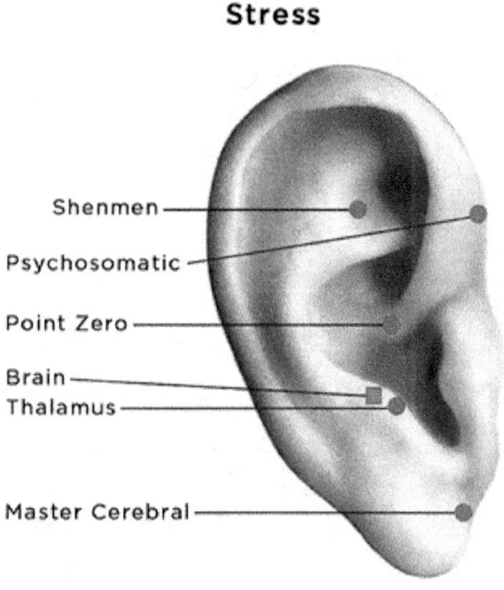

The Reverse Spin:

1) See if you can find where you store the discomfort. Give it a numerical value (1-10).

2) Locate the direction in which it's moving (it's always moving about inside).

3) Mimic the movement and slowly bring the rotation outside your body so it's in front of you.

4) Reverse the movement and slowly bring "it" back into your body.

5) Locate where the discomfort is now and, if you can, give it a numerical value.

6) Repeat until the discomfort is either gone or far more tolerable

Chapter 17:

Reclaiming Control of the Mind

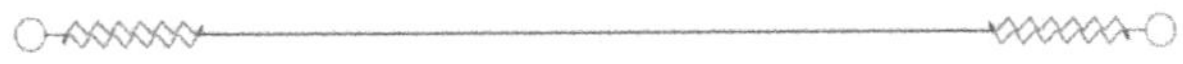

When the Sleep Wagon Is Wobbly

You've been using the tools I've laid out and followed the guidelines. The upshot has been positive: your stress and anxiety levels are down, and you are sleeping better than you had been. As a result, you feel great, and this improved state lasts a while. Suddenly, and without apparent reason — or perhaps there is a real reason--the wheels come off the sleep wagon, and you fall off it. What worked before no longer does. The mind is doing gerbil-like gyrations, and you're confused, angry and depressed. You want to climb back on the wagon, but nothing you do seems to work.

It's natural that you might ask, 'What happened!' In truth, temporary regression is not uncommon. We know the human mind is highly complex, and that its approach to itself is non-linear at best. Couple that with all of the daily stressors of life, and it's little wonder that sleep can again wobble on its axis. What to do?

The great news is that you have options. You've got breath work, Autogenic Training, the Staircase — the tools that helped in the past. You can also elevate your game using trance, or self-hypnosis.

When we talk about insomnia, what we're actually talking about is the mind misplacing its ability to create a positive future.

Insomnia roots you in past fears; in a conviction that since you didn't sleep recently, you probably won't sleep now or in the future. Your neural networks are stuck. But as we've seen, the seemingly simple act of imagining we're taking an action (remember the musician mentally practicing the arpeggio) can be a first step in helping you to build a new neural network.

Trance opens up networks to our future ability to rest and sleep well. By creating *new* behavior that is reflective of a future self, and specific time points in the future — a week, a month, three months — we're creating new neural networks that connect emotions, beliefs, and accomplishments. Infusing yourself with these future experiences can change the chemicals that flood your body. We then create physical anchors to hardwire them in muscle memory.

Erika

The insomnia had begun two years earlier, after a difficult breakup with a married man. During our initial intake, Erika shared that she was mired in alternating feelings of loss and rage, which tended to flare up at night. She had been to a talk therapist, and talking things out had helped, to a degree. She hoped hypnosis could help her shift her perspective, which was now negative, toward a more positive one.

 "I've got to get rid of that ghost that's still haunting my brain," she said with emphasis.

After making sure that she was a candidate for trance, we began with "future work". I used a V-A-K rich vision of her future where she was sleeping through the night, waking refreshed and free of her 'ghost." With each successive session, we reinforced the tools she would need. (see: Six Foundation Stones of Self-esteem in the next section). We then switched to acupuncture to strengthen her embattled nervous system and to embolden her on an emotional level. As Erika saw her old tendencies to self-sabotage in a new light, she began taking positive actions. Within six weeks she was sleeping again, and no longer feeling doomed if she happened to have an off night. We're now working on Erika's IBS which, not so coincidentally, has plagued her ever since the affair ended.

What Is Trance (aka self-hypnosis, or guided visualization)?

We all drift through multiple states of awareness on any given day. We may enter a state that we call "trance" without even knowing it. When we're immersed in a book, it's a form of trance. When we're lost in thought driving on a freeway and miss an exit, that too, is trance. The flickering TV screen mesmerizes us. When playing sports or being "in the zone" — even meditating — they're all on a continuum. Given that they all share a sense of focused awareness and relaxation, perhaps we can think of trance as availability for an altered experience.

History of Trance

Hypnosis first appeared 4,000 years ago, in the ancient city of Saqqara, in Egypt. An ailing citizen would speak with a priest/doctor concerning her problem. After undergoing a ritual cleansing, she would enter a darkened room within a sleep temple. There, under the rhythmic chanting of unseen voices, and mood-altering herbs, she would enter a state of trance.

Solutions to her problem would be offered and her responses acknowledged; a dialogue that might include forays into her dream world could go on for a number of hours. At a given point, she would emerge with a solution to her problem in place. This structured ritual lasted in Egypt for a thousand years before spreading to Greece, where it thrived for another millennium.

Hypnosis, as it came to be called, regained traction in the eighteenth century with Franz Mesmer. Sigmund Freud was an early devotee. It took another psychiatrist, Milton Erickson, to modernize hypnosis. By applying his skills of observation to the workings of the subconscious, he often helped people otherwise deemed beyond hope. Several researchers attempted to codify Erickson's brilliant, if opaque methods, and Neuro-Linguistic Programming is a pragmatic, if intuition-free result of that work.

Question: Is trance, or hypnosis, dangerous?

Answer: It's no more dangerous than relaxing into a wonderful nap.

Trance Today

If we want a picture of where trance exists today, we need look no further than Madison Avenue. The bright flickering tube amid the low chanting of commercials tells us what to eat, where to shop, and how our bodies should look if we want to fit into that expensive pair of jeans. The drip-drip from TV into our subconscious mind is a form of trance on a mass scale. But just as Madison Avenue can borrow our subconscious mind, we can seize it back. The first step is potentially the easiest: deciding how we want to be. In part, this entails consciously creating a reality that reflects our personal truth. Toward that end, I work with hypnosis clients using the Six Foundation Stones of Self-Esteem. They are:

1. Living Consciously

2. Being Assertive

3. Taking Self-responsibility

4. Personal Integrity

5. Having a Purpose (this is a big topic which I will address in another volume)

6. Self-Acceptance.

If you haven't yet formed an affirmation, do so now. Place it in the present tense. You're now ready to embed it into your subconscious mind, where it will do the most good. We do this in one of two ways. In the first method, you'll use familiar tools.

Method I:

(Affirmation)>Progressive Muscle Relaxation (or Autogenic Training)> The Staircase> Your Special Place.

The second one is the Betty E. Self-Hypnosis Method. This method entails using skills of observation.

Exercise 15: The Betty E. Self-Hypnosis Method

Listen to a recording of the Betty E Self-Hypnosis Method at rewiredforsleep.com/the-deeper-levels.

Betty, the wife of the aforementioned Doctor Erickson, was behind much of the advancement of modern-day trance, and it was she who developed this system for self-hypnosis that bears her name. The genius behind this deceptively simple method lies in its use of the V-A-K Sensor to help affirmations sink effortlessly into the subconscious.

Getting Started

1. Sit in a comfortable chair and take long, slow breaths, allowing your body to relax.

2. Determine a time limit — twenty minutes is standard, but it can be fifteen or thirty minutes.

3. State the affirmation out loud or silently. For instance: "I'm entering trance, and my unconscious mind helps me ____ (example: sleep through the night)." Alternately, you can write the affirmation on a slip of paper, read it to yourself, and then put the paper away. Include no more than two affirmations at any given time.

4. State how you want to feel at the end of the session, and then reinforce your affirmation. For example: "When I emerge in twenty minutes, I feel refreshed and revitalized, and ready to sleep through the night."

Affirmations on Sleep:

1. "I'm deeply relaxed and at night, head into a peaceful, restful sleep."

2. "I'm now entering into self-trance and easily sleep through the night. If I wake early, I can take three deep breaths and effortlessly go back to sleep."

Anxiety:

"I'm now entering self-trance so my unconscious mind can help me eliminate anxiety. When I return to the room, taking three deep breaths helps me feel peaceful and relaxed."

Entering into Self-Trance (V-A-K)

Get in a comfortable position, seated or lying down. Take three deep breaths; as you exhale, imagine a ripple of relaxation starting at the top of your head, and waving down to the bottom of your feet.

Part I (The External Section)

1. (V) Notice three objects. Go slowly, pausing briefly on each one. They can be small, such as a doorknob, lamp, or an item on the table. Some people name the items as they look at them. If any random thoughts float into your awareness, imagine them popping like bubbles. Don't try to completely still your mind. The system will work even if you feel scattered, or preoccupied.

2. (A) Turn your attention to what you hear. Notice three sounds: a clock ticking, a fan blowing, the creak of a settling building, cars passing by outside. Notice the sound of your breathing or make a sound by tapping your foot or clacking your teeth. If a noise was momentary, replay it in your head a few times.

3. (K) Shift your attention to your body; notice three sensations. Again, go slowly. Focus on sensations that normally are outside of your awareness, such as the weight of your eyeglasses, or the watch on your wrist, a piece of jewelry, article of clothing, the soles of your shoes, or the feel of your lips touching. You can even focus on an itch if you feel one.

4. Repeat this using two different objects, two different sounds, and two different feelings.

5. Repeat the cycle using one different object, one different sound, and one different feeling. At this point, you've completed the external portion of the process.

Part II: The Internal Section

Here you'll imagine an object, a sound and a sensation (using V-A-K). Close your eyes.

1. V: Imagine one small physical object. Perhaps it's a leaf, bird, or mirror. Focus your attention on the object for a minute or two.

2. A: Imagine one sound. It could be part of a song, or a train's whistle, or running water. Although this is the internal section, you can use an external sound if one comes to mind.

3. K: Imagine a single sensation. Maybe it's the warmth of the sun on your cheek, cool sand between your toes, a kiss on the lips, a comb across your scalp. Focus on it as if it were happening. If a physical sensation comes to your attention, you can use it.

4. Repeat the process with two different images, two different sounds, and two different feelings.

5. Repeat the cycle using three different images, three different sounds, and three different feelings.

That's it. If you do this exercise in the daytime, open your eyes and go about your business. If you've gone a little over your time or under it, don't worry. Practice yields better results. You may notice a profound change, or it might be subtle. Either way, I invite you to be grateful for even small shifts that your mind is making at all times to benefit you.

Chapter 18:

Barbara is a Punk Wiccan (Paradoxical Insomnia)

B arbara, 62, strikes a formidable image in a black jumpsuit, red motorcycle jacket, and beaded mandala necklace. She identifies as Wiccan (my intake form doesn't ask for religious affiliation) and suffers with longstanding fibromyalgia. But that isn't why she's in my office.

> "It's that sleep study they put me through," she says, with barely controlled anger.

That, and the resulting diagnosis: Paradoxical Insomnia, or a faulty perception of her own sleep. There is little Western medicine can do for it short of a prescription for anti-psychotic drugs.

> "Tests say I sleep better than I think I do," she says. "Forget them. I haven't had a decent night's rest in months! And they've got zilch for it except drugs. I mean, really?"

> Barbara's case is not so unique as one might think. Studies show that many people with sleep challenges are inaccurate in estimating the amount of sleep they get. They often overestimate the time it takes to fall asleep while underestimating total sleep time compared to objective brain-wave sleep recordings.

In a study in at the Stanford University sleep Clinic, 122 people with paradoxical insomnia spent the night in a sleep lab so that their sleep could be measured with brain-wave recordings. On average, these individuals overestimated the time it took them to fall asleep by thirty minutes and underestimated total sleep time by one hour. One reason for this is that insomniacs incorrectly perceive light stages of sleep, such as Stage 2 sleep, as wakefulness. However, recall that Stage 2 sleep is a valid sleep stage. Adults spend half the night and the elderly most of the night in this stage.

I know that there's little be gained by trying to tell Barbara that she's getting more sleep than she thinks she is. We use acupuncture, which can start the process of unwinding her Sympathetic Nervous System. Later, we'll add herbs, along with other modalities, so long as she is open to them. One is Neuro-Linguistic Programming, and My Friend John/Jane exercise.

My Friend John/Jane

In utilizing "My Friend Jane," Barbara steps outside of herself in order to help another person I ask Barbara how she'd help a friend ("Jane"). She replies effortlessly, seeming to surprise even herself.

1. Define the problem: *I don't know what to do with myself.*

2. Clarify the goal(s): *I could take time out to clear my head.*

3. Generate solutions: *Take a walk, come back and hang out with my cat, Ponzi. Try not to isolate.*

4. Experiment with new solutions: *Call my old friend, Sonya, and say* *hello.*

"I read that Chinese doctors used to give their patients exercises," Barbara says. "Let's do it!"

I give Barbara printouts for Six Healing Sounds and Autogenic Training. When I see her again, she tells me she's taking a Qi Gong class and loving every minute of it. "I swear," she says, "I think it's helping my fibro". She has also gotten in touch with her old friend, Sonya, who has an essential oils business. Barbara buys a starter kit and is soon blending them. She places essential oils on different acupoints and then records her bodily responses to them in minute detail. Frankly, I applaud Barbara's inner mad scientist. She is on a mission to take charge of her health, even if it means going outside her comfort zone to do so.

What are Essential Oils?

Nearly every major culture from antiquity to the present has used essential oils for one purpose or another. The pleasing aroma aside, they can change mood, calm, or even invigorate. Some people place them under their pillow, while others get a diffuser and imbue a room with a scent of their choosing. The following essential oils are often used for sleep issues. Note: Due to their potency, essential oils can potentially be harmful for children and pregnant women. Never take essential oils internally. Use a carrier oil for topical use.

- Bergamot comes from the peel of a citrus fruit and reduces anxiety and depression. Note: Bergamot is photosensitive. Avoid applying before going outside or apply to covered skin.

- Chamomile has a light, floral scent and creates a peaceful ambience in your bedroom.

- Lavender: The oil may be used as a compress, massage oil, or inhaled. You can also place a few drops under your pillowcase at night (use 10 drops essential oil per ounce of vegetable oil), or 3-5 drops in baths.

- Jasmine has sedative characteristics, making it useful for insomnia, stress, and fatigue.

- Neroli is said to have anti-depressant qualities and calms the nervous system.

- Sandalwood helps remedy insomnia, anxiety, and tension

Topical Use: Apply at bedtime to sleep points Anmian, Yintang, and Shimian (a new point)

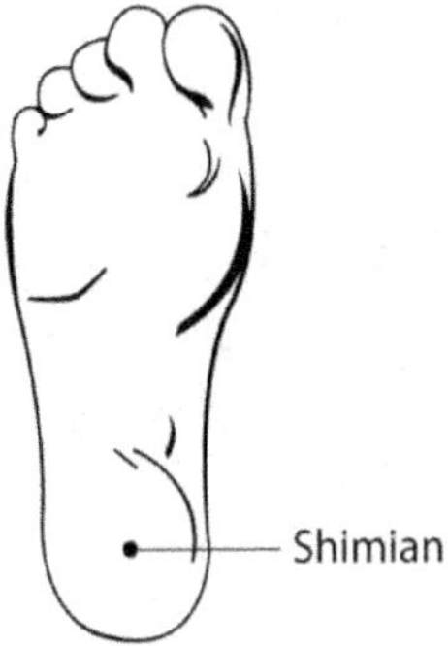

Shimian (Difficulty Sleeping) is a special point for sleep. Massage or use a Tiger Warmer.

I tell Barbara that acupuncture isn't magic, and it can take time before sleep kicks in. Nevertheless, at her next session, she lets me know she is unhappy. It's true that her sleep has improved, but not to her satisfaction. Before I can say that the body's got its own timetable for healing, Barbara says:

"Why don't we try hypnosis. I know my negative attitudes aren't doing me any good."

After discussing the process with her, and checking to see that she is a candidate, I relax her fully.

Normally, I know precisely how I will direct a session, and what I will say. Once in a while, however, I allow something else to occur. I liken it to how a jazz musician feels when they're "in the pocket" with other musicians, or when an athlete is "in the zone". I start by relaxing Barbara while keeping her mind sharp. As subtle signs that she is in an altered state appear, this time I allow for my unconscious to become engaged in the process.

"You know, science has determined that our universe has up to eleven dimensions rather than the three we are in touch with. It's entirely possible that, in another dimension, you're always awake, just as you say you are." I briefly wonder whether I've crawled too far out on this limb; having decided to trust the process, I press on. "You're just confusing your dimensions, which is understandable given that we've got eleven of them."

She slowly nods her head in agreement.

"And isn't it good to know, that, in this dimension, you can sleep through the night."

I continue to direct my words to her subconscious mind, offering Barbara multiple choices:

"I don't know whether you'll sleep tonight, or tomorrow night...or perhaps the night after that. You may choose to sleep through the night later this week. And isn't it good to have a choice when you'll sleep."

Soon after I emerge Barbara from her state of relaxation, she pays, and exits stage right.

At her next session, Barbara grabs hold of my hand and shakes it forcefully.

"Whatever the hell you did," she says, "that night I slept for the first time in months."

"You did all the work," is my honest reply. "All I did was show you the door; you walked through it."

Barbara signs on for what she calls 'the Cadillac treatment": Hypnopuncture.

As its name implies, this modality entails using hypnosis and acupuncture at the same time. If the word 'synergy' has been worn to the nub, it is applicable to hypnopuncture for certain difficult cases. This is especially true in the arena of sleep, anxiety, and symptoms associated with IBS. I don't mean to imply that Chinese medicine alone isn't an effective stand-alone protocol for these issues, because it is. But there is much to be said for aligning acupuncture with the power of trance work that, beyond the elegance of melding two seemingly different systems, yields results that often are deeply effective.

During our next session, I insert seven pins along Barbara's arms and legs, and we begin. I mentally direct her to descend an escalator to a corridor, and to a door with a sign that says, "Sleep room." I ask her to open the door and then tell me what she sees. Barbara finds herself in a lighted cave. There is a bearskin rug that serves as a blanket; on a table there's a cooked veal shank and a bottle of Rioja, and nearby, a hearth, with a cozy fire. After finishing her meal, she snuggles under the bearskin blanket and sees herself heading off to slumber. In this way, Barbara has created a pathway that leads to the doors of sleep.

A week later Barbara comes in. She doesn't even mention the issue of sleep, which surprises me, in a good way.

"The Qi Gong helped my fibromyalgia, but I'm still in pain. I leave for Paris in two weeks. Can you just fix it before I go? Come on Doc, you're good."

"Thanks for the vote of confidence," I reply, trying to maintain a straight face, "but fibromyalgia's considered a chronic disease. Even using Chinese medicine, it can take many months to resolve. Besides, diet is crucial, which means none of those yummy French desserts. Can you commit to that?"

"Ha! Not on your life!" She suddenly becomes wistful: "You know, over the last few weeks, I'm able to sleep sometimes. I even wake up feeling almost refreshed."

Given Barbara's old investment in the no-sleep story, I consider this modified assessment a sign of progress. There are times when both healer and patient need to be grateful for even small steps forward. I suggest Barbara take Vitamin D3 for the fibromyalgia, and that she start doing the Microcosmic Orbit in order to move energy through the blockages to help relieve the pain. Of course, she can always use a Tiger Warmer on TW3,). LI4), SI3 and the relevant points found on the auricular chart.

As a follow up, Barbara has become enamored of essential oils. She and her old friend, Sonya, are now repping a well-known line. Barbara has ditched her neo-punk look and is now sporting thigh-high suede boots and matching hat, and a pricey poncho. She is also a fount of information about EO's, as they're called, and I wish her well on her new business venture. I demur when she invites me out to lunch with Sonya.

PART II

Perchance to Sleep:

Rewiring the Circuits

*"Put your thoughts to sleep, do not let them cast a shadow
over the moon of your heart.*

Let go of thinking."

– Rumi

The following case histories showcase how various patients responded to treatment. If the methods appear opaque at times, that's because I've compressed them for the sake of brevity. My goal is to demonstrate the tools at your disposal; as always, it's up to you to find the combination of methods that work best for you.

Helene uses Stomach 36), magnolia bark, Move the Voice, Meridian Tapping, along with two new points, CV17 and DU20.

Jeffrey Runs PTSD Down (Maintenance Insomnia): Auricular Protocol for PTSD; affirmations, Abdominal breathing, Autogenic Training, Staircase>Special Place; Butterfly Hug and short form Tapping.

Annabelle: (Onset Insomnia): Move the Voice, Reverse Spin; Kava and Restore Spleen Decoction; Tiger Warmer on ST36).; Five, Five, and Five.

Margaret: Treats menopausal symptoms with acupuncture and herbs.

Raymond's Path: A program for weaning oneself from sleep medication in a responsible manner.

Pediatric Acupressure: Strengthen your child's immune system with acupressure.

Helene: Phoenix Rises from the Ashes, and Flies

"Anxiety's always been with me," says Helene. She is the feisty magazine editor whom we first met in the preface to this book. "My shrink says perfectionism, bulimia, and career achievement held it at bay. Then it all went to hell in LA. I know, it's my fault for crapping where I eat."

What she is referring to in vivid manner is an affair with a Twitter-happy subordinate, the souring of which imploded on social media. A problem with sleep and digestion blew up into diagnoses of IBS, insomnia, and depression. Since her return to New York, she has been plowing through doctors. It appears I am next in line. If being the proverbial caboose on the physician train is a status that most acupuncturists know too well, it's one that many of us have come to relish, rather than resent.

Helene pulls up her iconic T-Rex tee-shirt to reveal her abdomen.

"My belly," she exclaims, "is massively distended. The GI says my IBS is incurable. What say you?"

"I'd say your GI Doctor is wrong. Now, let's do some hypnopuncture."

We do two sessions of hypnopuncture within three days of each other.

A week later, Helene comes in and excitedly shows me her suddenly flat belly. There's nothing magical about bloating going down, of course. That said, she uses it as leverage to further ignite her self-repair process. Helene picks up a Tiger Warmer and moxa sticks and starts using them on Spleen 9 and Stomach 36 (ST36).. Known to benefit digestion and the immune system,

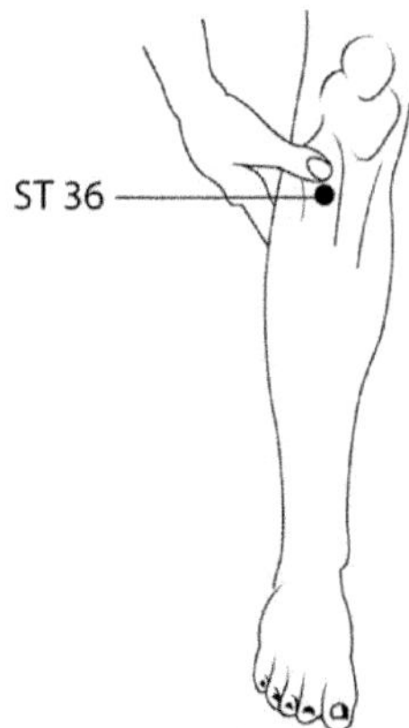

moxa on ST36 is used by Elderly Chinese men to increase longevity and vitality.

I prescribe for Helene Magnolia bark in pill form to further relieve bloating. If Helene is impatient for faster progress, she also sees how far she has come and is hungry for more of the same.

That said, it is her relationship with her mother that, pushes her "buttons" like nobody's business.

I suggest we use "Move the Voice" to diminish the power of Mom.

"Is this more of your pop psychology," she says, half-grousing, but clearly engaged.

"Close your eyes for a minute," I say. "Imagine that Mom is haranguing you."

"That's a stretch."

"Where in your head is her voice? Upper, lower, left, right?",

"Right upper quadrant."

"Now, you mentioned that your dad treated you …"

"Like the princess that I am."

"Can you hear his voice?"

"Lower left side. Cool as an October breeze."

"Place her voice in that lower left, cooler quadrant."

Helene becomes quiet for a minute.

"She's lost her piss and vinegar. For now, anyway. Not bad."

In the next session we Tap on anxiety. (See Extra Mile 1.5: Tapping for Anxiety protocol.)

After the first round, Helene's anxiety levels rose from a "6" to a "9." That's not uncommon. The anxious mind often pushes back in an effort to maintain what it perceives as necessary control.

We do two more sequences in rapid succession.

"Tell me what level the discomfort is at now."

"It's down," she replies flatly, "from an eight to a three." She suddenly laughs and shakes her head in disbelief.

If there is one thing a catastrophist likes more than being right, it is having clear evidence that she will not, in fact, fall off the face of the earth.

Acupuncture becomes Helene's treatment of choice, and she dives into it even more deeply.

At night, she does self-massage on CV17 and DU20. Conception Vessel 17, or CV17, is located at the center of the breast, three thumb widths up from the base of the bone and between the nipples. It helps relieve insomnia caused by anxiety and chest congestion. Rotate two fingers twenty-four times in each direction while taking deep breaths. Do not use moxa on this point.

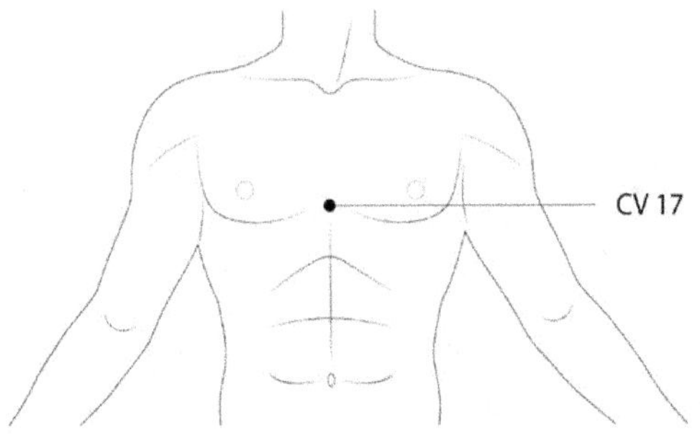

The other point, DU20 (Bai Hui, 100 Convergences) is also known as Top of Head point in Meridian Tapping. It's located on the midline of the head, roughly on the midpoint of the line connecting the tops of the two ears. The literature states that it helps to ease symptoms of insomnia and depression. Massage, or tap with the palm of the hand.

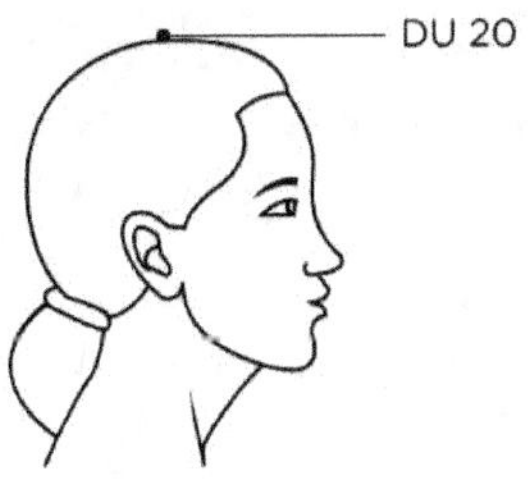

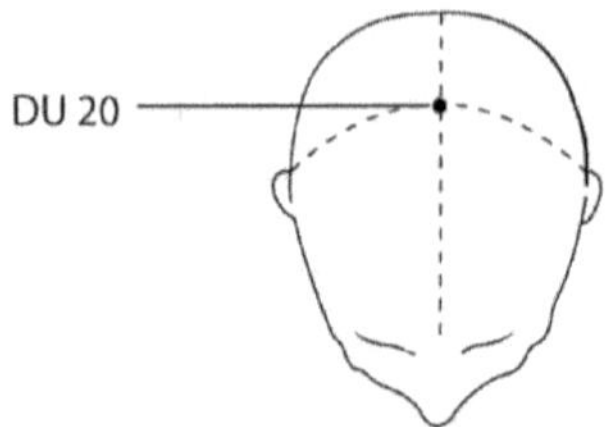

Helene struggles with depression and so uses the auricular protocol shown in the illustration below. She massages the ear seeds until they fell off, at which point she replaces them. "It's the

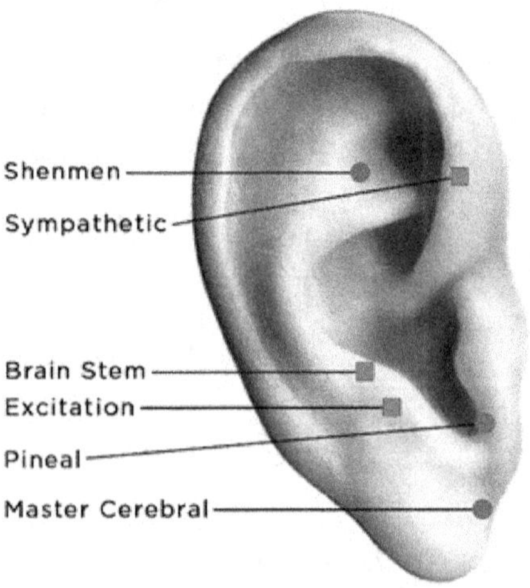

damnedest thing," Helene says, "the seeds really calm me down in a pinch."

Helene has decided to ditch Seroquel, a medicine for depression that she's been taking. She assures me that she has cleared this important step with her psychiatrist.

"What's at stake," she says, "is fear versus taking back my power, once and for all. It's letting go of mom, once and for all. This is my line in the sand, pure and simple."

The psychiatrist takes a dim view of Chinese herbs but permits Helene to take St. John's Wort, a Western herb, for the depression. The detox process entails removing grains from her capsules on an incremental basis. She does this for several months, but can't seem to get past fifty percent without her digestive system going haywire. Finally, it seems, she is over the proverbial hump. She is thrilled.

"I'm noticing an improvement in my overall mood," Helene tells me. "It's spinning class."

"It must be that," I reply. Her endorphins truly deserve all the credit.

"Forget Los Angeles," she says, perhaps more to herself than to me. "My life's still ahead of me, I've just got to decide how to live it."

Helene is writing again, but she will no longer do fluff pieces. Despite her love of the world of publishing, she's given up her apartment in New York and is moving to Fairfield, Connecticut in order to be closer to nature, and to the ocean. We continue doing monthly hypnosis sessions by Skype.

Jeffrey Runs PTSD Down (Maintenance Insomnia)

Jeffrey, a 31-year-old African American, wakes up at 2 a.m. like clockwork, his mind racing and body shaking with fear. Maintenance insomnia, as interrupted sleep is called, is among the most common sleep disorders, and Jeffrey's amygdala-based response often means he is done sleeping for the night. Being a pharmaceutical rep, Jeffrey is always talking to doctors and writing reports. He is also a self-avowed gym rat with chronic shoulder pain at the deltoid and subscapularis muscles. The problems, he tells me, began when he was in the army.

> "Life got real on that first tour. I stopped sleeping. It wasn't till I was back home in Jersey City for a while that I was able to make it through the night in one piece. Then I got redeployed. Couple of my buds didn't make it back, and...it's called survivor's guilt, right? I didn't think it was real, until ..."

Jeffrey clears his throat and fidgets in the chair. Sadness floats through the shiny onyx pebbles of his eyes.

"When did the insomnia kick in?"

"Before the, ah, psychotic episode. They sent me home. The dreams do some nasty numbers on my head. I got a shrink for that."

"Meds?"

"Anti-psychotics, and Ambien so I could sleep. Weaned myself off both."

"I give you credit. Kicking Ambien alone can be pretty tough."

"I sell that shit, so I know the side effects. I just need to sleep. So ...can you help me?"

"That's what I'm here for. Ever been diagnosed with PTSD?"

"Yeah. I didn't think anything could help that."

"We'll start there."

Auricular PTSD Protocol

The roots of Post-Traumatic Stress Disorder, or PTSD, can be traced to soldiers who had experienced trauma during wartime. More currently, the term is used to describe the effects of traumatic events with either emotional or physical basis.

This is the PTSD auricular protocol we used for Jeffrey:

Auricular Trauma Protocol (ATP)

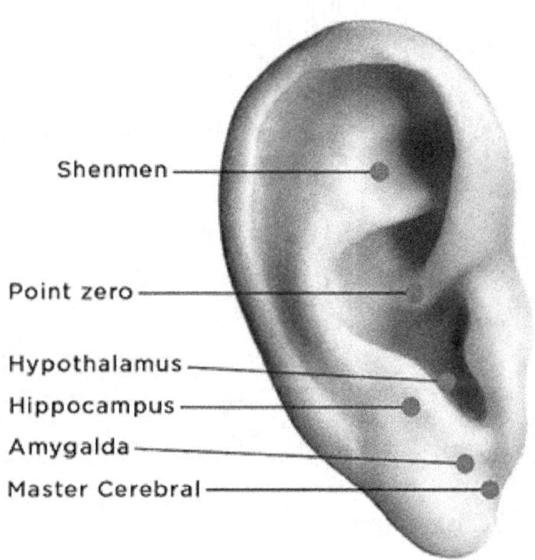

Shenmen: Spirit Gate. Alleviates pain: acupoints and anxiety, depression, insomnia and stressful states.

Point Zero: Helps reboot the body to a state of homeostatic balance; relieves spasms.

Hypothalamus: Stimulates the parasympathetic functions of calming and anxiety control.

Hippocampus: Influences memory encoding and concentration.

Amygdala: Modulates irritability, anger, fear, and aggression.

Master Cerebral: Influential in chronic pain. The prefrontal cortex zone is located there.

After four treatments, Jeffrey's shoulder is ninety percent better. He decides this is a perfect time to hit the gym again, and is soon back in my office.

> "I don't mind the cycle of pain," he says, before I can give him my pitch to cut back, "as long as I can keep working out."

Jeffrey formulates a repair plan in his sleep journal. Here is how he breaks down the process:

1. Affirmation: "I am a creature of God filled with love that I embody freely.

2. Abdominal Breathing, followed by Autogenic Training.

3. After listening to a recording of the Staircase, I visualize going through a door into:

4. My Special Place: a beachfront condo in Negril, Jamaica.

By this point, Jeffrey is often fast asleep.

If he wakes up in the middle of the night, he does Butterfly Hug and Rain Forest meditation (found in Extra Mile 1.5).

Because of Jeffrey's PTSD, his Sympathetic Nervous System is still prone to being overloaded at the smallest sensory stimuli. To help counteract it, I show him what I've termed, "Short form Tapping."

Short Form Tapping

Since it may feel disruptive to do Meridian Tapping in the middle of the night, I've created a shortened version utilizing just four points on the hand. One of them, Pericardium 8 (PC8), is a new point. Aside from easing nausea and anxiety, PC8 is considered a fulcrum point on the body for energy. I use it for sleep issues, as it is a hand mirror-image point to one on the sole of the foot, Kidney 1 (KI1). Find it at the tip of your middle finger when you make a fist.

[Note: using pressure, or moxa with Tiger Warmer, on PC8 and KI-1, in succession, is particularly helpful for treating sleep issues.]

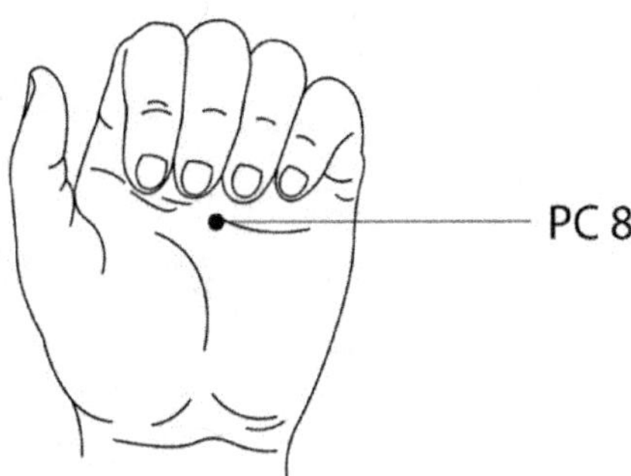

Jeffrey places his left hand in his right and taps PC8, PC6), HT7), and TW3.

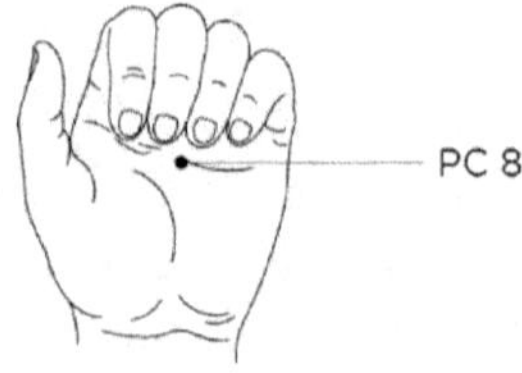

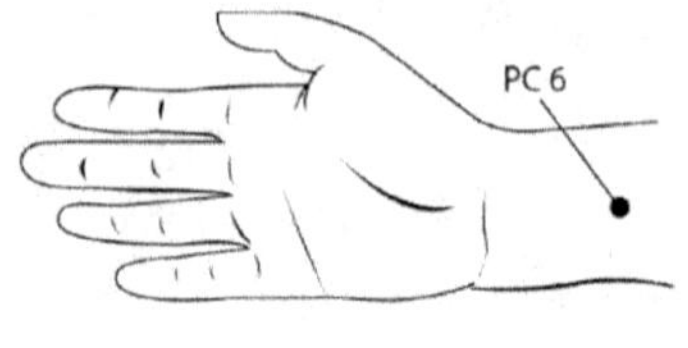

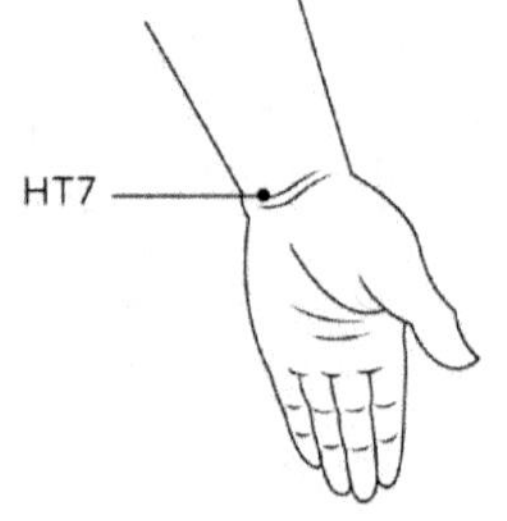

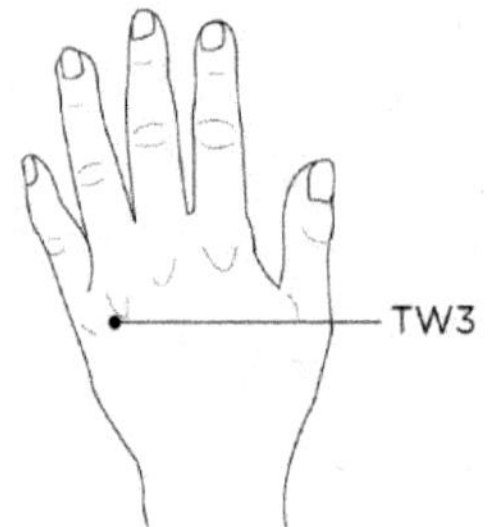

To go with compressed Tapping, we simplify the verbal part as well.

"Sleep and let go."

"Sleep, accept."

"Sleep easy."

"Letting go, now."

Exercise 16: Desensitize Touch Protocol for Pain

Pain is considered to be a subjective response, meaning we can have a measure of control over it. Typically, an effort to ignore it does little other than to make it more pronounced. But we can often lessen its impact by focusing on the sensation rather than trying to ignore it. To do this, we bring back our old friend, The Pauli Principle (no two objects can occupy the same physical space) to explain Desensitize Touch Protocol. In this context, we diminish an unwanted sensation by duplicating it.

1. Bring your awareness to the area of discomfort. Rate it on a scale of 1 to 10 (10 being worst).

2. Starting five inches from the center of the discomfort, slowly move your finger toward it in a circular pattern. Touch the area around it over the course of a minute or even longer.

3. See if the pain has changed. Now move your finger away in a slow, circular pattern.

4. Repeat the process several times. The discomfort may move, lessen, or even disappear.

Note: When it comes to pain, always have it checked out by an MD.

It is Jeffrey's modus operandi to push himself in everything he does. It's unfortunate that his workouts and shoulder discomfort reflect this single-mindedness. I show him the auricular Pain module, and the shoulder point on the ear, and he starts using a Tiger Warmer to positive effect. Seeking greater flexibility, he joins a Hatha Yoga class, where he meets Kendra, a part-time instructor there. In time he sees how weightlifting is not serving his needs and, reluctantly at first, he lets go the routine. His shoulder improves further. His PTSD also eases. It doesn't hurt that he is spending time with Kendra.

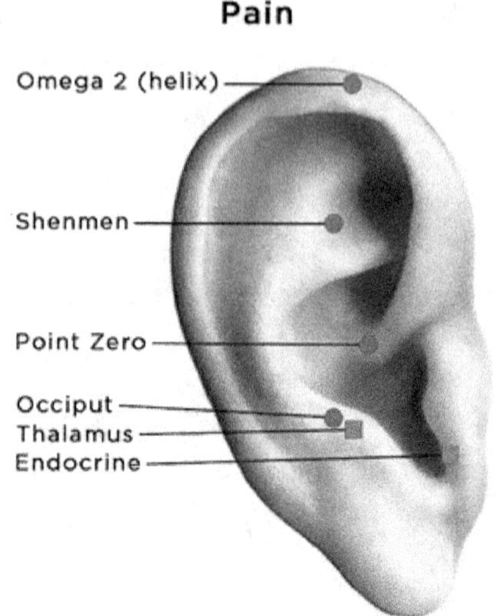

Jeffrey gets a promotion at work, but stability finds him in other ways: he and Kendra have gotten engaged. He is also playing piano again, which he gave up at age eleven due to family finances. Jeffrey is now composing music for meditation.

"Down the road, I want this to be my main source of income. Kendra's a nurse's aide, but she's also a singer, and she's down with that idea, too."

Case of The Sleep-Disturbed Leopard (Onset Insomnia)

Annabelle, 34, is wiry, with a shy smile and gray eyes that lock on you like lasers. She has been struggling with insomnia for fourteen months, has chronic anxiety, and stress-induced diarrhea. Above her right ear, where her head is shaved is an exquisitely inked spotted leopard in mid-pounce.

"I'm okay once I'm asleep," she says. "But the next day I'm exhausted, almost as if I'd run a marathon. That's called Onset Insomnia, right?"

"That's right." It's also a diagnosis that offers no solutions. It's my job to decipher what will in fact, help her sleep. With her next question, it seems she has read my mind.

"How do you know what'll work for me?"

"We observe, ask questions. I'd check whether the anxiety is based in the amygdala or in the prefrontal cortex."

"Amygdala-based here. Always been anxious, but my mom's diagnosis of pancreatic cancer last year kicked it up. Ever since she died, I've had non-stop racing thoughts at night."

Acupuncture is my opening gambit, and Annabelle takes to it, committing to twice weekly treatments.

As a bookkeeper for a small, start-up tech firm, she works from home so she can have more time for her three-year-old daughter, while also juggling a song writing career.

"I'm grateful for the gig," she says during her third session. "But my boss is a jerk. He makes unrealistic demands on me, and that kicks up all sorts of fear. At times it feels as though I can hardly breathe."

I listen but say nothing. The second time she raises the same topic, we do Reverse Spin.

Annabelle and the Reverse Spin

"Where in your body is the anxiety?" I say. "Take a moment to locate it."

Her hands hover over her heart before descending to the area around her liver. She is feeling around for the discomfort, finally locating it in her lower abdomen.

"Give it a numerical value," I say. "Ten being bad."

"Nine. Wait! It's in my side now. Oh, man, so angry. Old shit. Right here."

Annabelle rotates her arm before her in a widening orbit, then reverses the spin and moves it back inside her body.

"What number is it now?" I say.

"Soft five." She sounds unsure.

"You feel it anywhere else?"

Pointing to her upper chest, Annabelle moves her hand forward in a widening arc. She soon puts her whole her body into it, rotating her arm fiercely, like a crazed harpist wind-milling her instrument. Finally, she reverses the spin, brings her hand to her chest, and comes to a full stop.

"What number is it now?"

"I can't locate it," she replies.

I leave the room in order to give Annabelle time to gather herself. When I return, there is a perplexed grin on her face.

"Craziest thing," she says. "I could see and feel all the anger, like a lifetime of garbage swirling around in me. Then, when I reversed the spin, the garbage suddenly changed into a field of daisies, and I felt … how can I say this: happy."

Kava's Fine, but …

I prescribe for Annabelle a tincture of Kava, an herb commonly used to ease anxiety. Some people find it is "heavy" on the body; others wouldn't function without having their beloved "Kava Kava."

"Not for me!" says Annabelle when I next see her. "It was like I've got cotton candy in my head. Given my life right now, it's more brain fuzz than I can handle." I laugh at the image of brain fuzz.

Because she runs cold, is prone to palpitations and has loose bowels, I give her Restore the Spleen Decoction an herb formula that addresses all three issues—and help with sleep as well.

"My new ritual is put Sam to bed, read her to sleep and then do self-care." Twice a week Annabelle uses a Tiger Warmer on Stomach 36, first on Sam and then on herself, adding Spleen 9 to treat her tendency toward loose bowels.

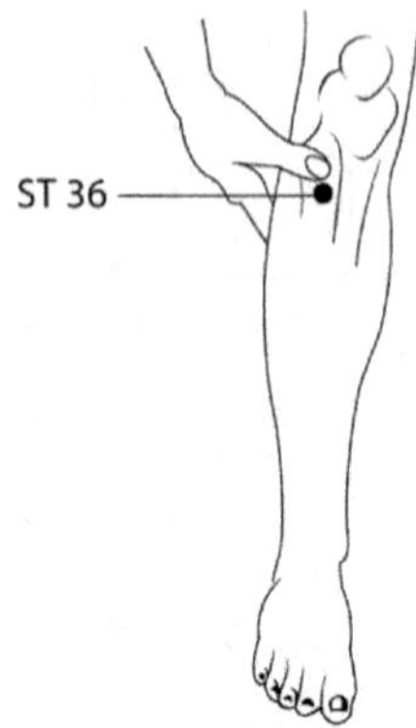

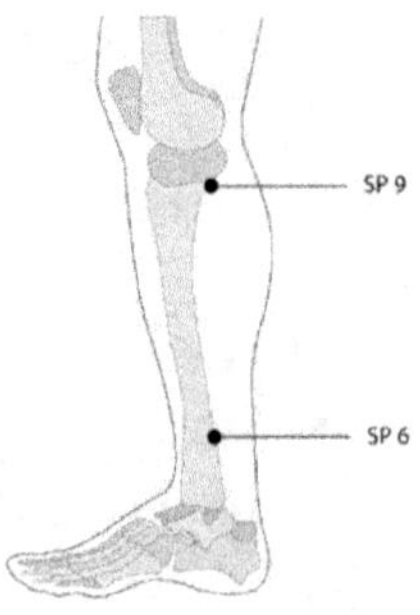

Annabelle also tapes ear seeds to the auricular digestive module and massages them daily.

Digestive Issues

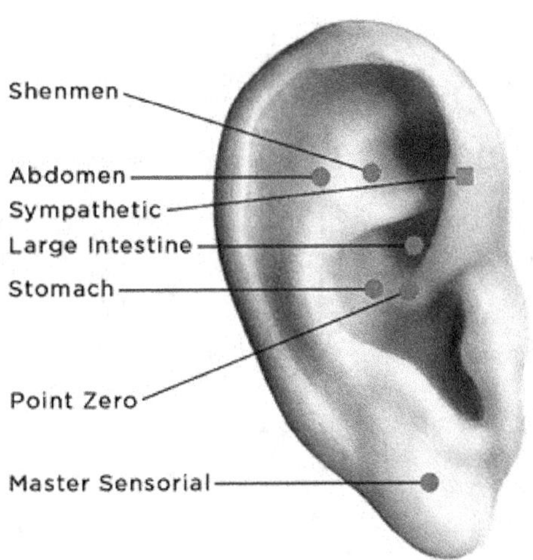

She also has started doing the Five, Five, and Five exercise nightly.

Consistency pays off: she is often asleep within twenty minutes of turning off the lights. If Sam climbs into her bed, Annabelle's there for her but then falls back asleep relatively quickly. This is what progress looks like. We leave the prospect of future sessions open-ended.

Three months later Annabelle comes in, complaining of a mild urinary tract infection.

"How have you been sleeping?" I ask, as I treat the UTI.

"I get seven hours, which is damn near awesome. And I'm still gunning for a full eight."

Ginger Rogers and the Hot Flash

"We didn't talk about depression," says Margaret in a savory Hungarian accent. "When you felt bad you just pulled yourself up and kept working. I don't sleep so good."

Her hooded eyelids are those of someone who grew up peering out from behind the folds of the iron curtain. The rust tone of her silk blouse matches her short, wavy hair. A closed Spanish fan in her hand tells me that menopause is taking a toll on this 55-year-old woman's ability to sleep through the night.

"It's like waves of heat wash over me," she says, flipping open her fan reflexively.

Margaret's symptoms are not uncommon. One in four peri-menopausal or menopausal women has trouble sleeping. The hormonal stew being churned up during this time of life can also be a factor in depression.

"I work my whole life taking care of my husband and three kids," she says, pride and bitterness wrapped together inextricably. "I also have shoulder pain, but it's nothing."

"There's a saying," I say, "about a movie dance couple, Ginger Rogers and Fred Astaire."

"I love Ginger Rogers."

"Then you'll know: Ginger did everything Fred did, but backwards and in high heels."

Margaret smiles politely. I needn't explain to her this metaphor for how women often navigate the workplace, working harder and jumping through smaller hoops than men do while carrying the burden of work at home. She has lived it.

"I think we can ease the heat and the shoulder pain. That alone ought to help you sleep." I insert eight thin pins just under Margaret's skin. I don't mention that Japanese medicine refers to a syndrome related to shoulder pain, called "fifty-year-old syndrome."

When she emerges from the treatment room, a calm demeanour has replaced the wary one.

"I feel different." She rotates her shoulder." And my neck feels looser. Light."

For homework, Margaret uses a Tiger Warmer on Kidney 6) and on Kidney 1.

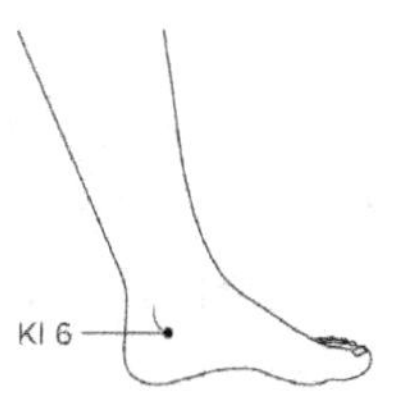

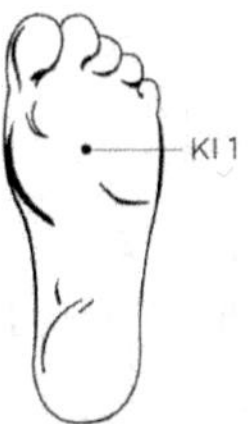

Margaret is open to Meridian Tapping for menopause, even if it strikes her as odd. (See Extra Mile 1.5 chapter for Meridian Tapping for Hot Flashes.)

I ask her to identify an emotion that has been bothering her.

"I am angry I don't speak up for myself. I'm afraid it's rubbed off on my daughters."

I prescribe for her Black Cohosh, an herb for hot flashes, and Wild Yam (Dioscorea villos), which is known for its active ingredient diosgenin, a phytoestrogen. Since low estrogen levels contribute to insomnia, I also give Margaret a list of foods that act as phytoestrogens.

Phytoestrogen Rich Food

Nuts and seeds: flaxseed, sunflower seeds, sesame seeds, almonds, and walnuts.

Fruits: Apples, carrots, pomegranates, strawberries, cranberries, and grapes.

Phytoestrogen rich vegetables include yams, lentils, alfalfa sprouts, mung beans, sprouts.

Subsequent acupuncture sessions ease her hot flashes. "I feel better, my shoulder is not a hundred percent," she confesses but adds that she is happy with the progress, even if I am not. Her elder daughter, who first found me online and struggles with IBS and sleep, is now a patient.

Raymond's Path: Detoxing from Sleep Aids

With his beet-red hair and gold stud earrings, Raymond, 33, would stand out even if he were not 6'6". As the head of an entertainment law firm he has a stable of known clients, some of whom even I recognize by name. His days are spent on the phone or reading contracts, and his nights at music venues pressing flesh. Seemingly boundless energy only adds to his commanding presence.

"I broke my left fibula skiing last year," he begins, sounding rushed, like he's late for a meeting. "The pain was crazy, so my primary gave me Vicodin. I liked how it made me feel. Too much. Trying to quit was brutal, and my husband almost left me. I spent a month rehabbing, then booze came in. When I quit that, I couldn't sleep, so it was hello, Xanax. I've got to sleep, if only for work."

"You have a history with medication?" I ask, still working on the intake. "It all stays here."

"When you're in the music biz people just assume all sorts of things about you. I went to Yale Law, Magna Cum Laude. Never even touched cough syrup, let alone drugs."

Raymond's addiction to pain pills is an all-too common story. The problem is made all that much worse by lack of monitoring on the part of the medical establishment. I've seen a ninety-four-year-old woman with Oxycodone in her system for surgery being released from a hospital and told to detox on her own. There is something wrong with a medical system that would allow anyone, let alone an elderly person, leave managed care without scheduling follow-ups for drug withdrawal.

Weaning Yourself Off Medication

If you've been taking sleep aids for over twenty-one days consecutively, you're better off not trying to stop outright. The prospect of rebound insomnia is as inevitable as the anxiety, headaches, fatigue, muscle spasms, and/or nausea that are its symptoms. Unmonitored Benzodiazepine withdrawal can lead to seizures.

That's why I urge you to enlist help from your doctor or other informed therapist, such as a Naturopath, acupuncturist, or psychiatrist. There's no universal treatment strategy for detoxing, but essential tools are self-acceptance, discipline and self-awareness. Along with the following tools, they will help mitigate your discomfort:

Tools for Detoxification.

1. Breath Work and Progressive Muscle Relaxation help to relax achy muscles.

2. Four-Step Trauma Intervention. Bi-lateral stimulation can help defuse anxiety.

3. Six Healing Sounds (Focus on Liver, Triple Burner, and Lung)

4. Meridian Tapping: Use the drug detox script found in Extra Mile, 1.5.

5. Butterfly Hug. Helps with feelings of pain, sadness, abandonment, fear.

6. Autogenic Training helps your control your heart rate, your breathing, your body.

7. Herbs: Kava for relaxation. Kudzu is an herb that eases the effects of toxicity.

8. Free and Easy Wanderer is a Chinese formula that can ease the nervous, anxious mind.

9. Acupoints. Many of the points we've accessed can be of help here. By symptom, they are:

A. Anxiety: LV3, CV17 and Yintang. Place your right middle fingertip at Yintang and your left hand on CV17. Apply medium pressure to both points for one minute while taking long, slow, deep breaths through your nostrils. LV3 is a point you can massage/Tiger Warmer at night.

B. Gastric problems: diarrhea or constipation. CV12 (Zhong Wan, or Central Stomach).

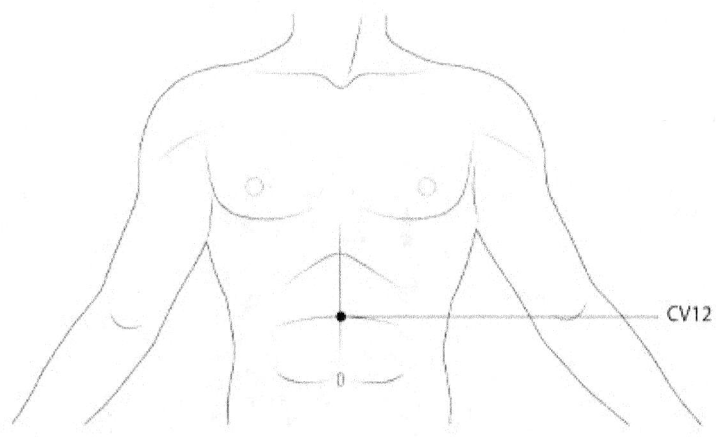

CV12 is located four finger inches above the umbilicus and is used for stomach ache, abdominal distention, nausea, vomiting, acid reflux, diarrhea, morning sickness, indigestion and insomnia. As usual, you can massage the point or use a Tiger Warmer. Another powerful point for any sort of GI problems is Stomach 36.

Soon after receiving my acupuncture license, I enrolled in a course on detox auriculotherapy at Lincoln Hospital, in the South Bronx. This was in 1996, and the crack epidemic in New York was in full swing. I took a part-time job at a group home for women whose children had been taken away from them due to drug use. Those tough, tender women were rooting for each other to stay clean, and I was too.

It's abundantly obvious that the dire situations of inner-city women differ radically from those of a product of white privilege. And yet, they all share a common reality: whether it's crack or

Ambien, detoxing is a form of hell. The image below shows the auricular protocol I used then, and that I still use as part of a larger protocol for helping people get off any chemical substance.

Drug Involvement

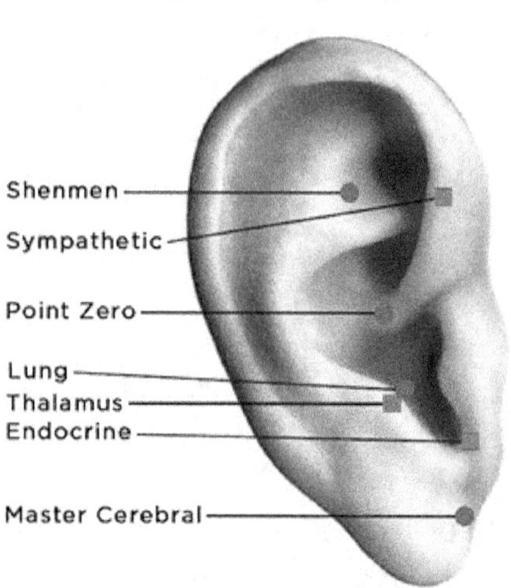

*Shenmen – Spirit Gate. Alleviates pain and anxiety, depression, insomnia and stressful states.

Sympathetic: Used to regulate SNS and PNS; Strong analgesic and relaxant effect.

*Point Zero: Helps reboot the body to a state of homeostatic balance; relieves spasms

Lung: Used for respiratory and skin illness; night sweats, anesthesia, cravings.

Thalamus: Over excitement, sweating, PTSD, fear, irritability.

Endocrine: Regulates disturbance of endocrine functions; the digestive system.

*Master Cerebral: Influential in chronic pain.

Keep it simple: Stimulate the points you can and leave the rest.

The Rewired Detox Program

Set a date when stressors in your life will be low, and then do your best to stick to a schedule.

Days 1–21: Take 7/8th of the full dosage.

Days 22–42: Take 3/4th of the full dosage.

Days 43–63: at 5/8ths.

Days 64–84 should be at 50% of the full dosage.

Continue at a 21-day pace to 3/8ths, and so on.

Note: This is a guideline only. When you are doing a stepwise detox, resist the temptation to take even one pill. Giving in to the "just this one pill will get me over the hump" mindset is a short hop back to full dosage. I urge you to take advantage of the aforementioned tools instead.

Aftermath: Raymond's path has proven to be, as he puts it, "twisty, at best." After putting himself, and his husband, through several harrowing slips involving pills and alcohol, he has regained his equilibrium and now is cautiously hopeful. Raymond is scheduled for root canal work and offered Vicodin for pain. This time, his husband takes control of the pills, doling them out to him on an as-needed basis. I too, am cautiously hopeful for Raymond. In any case, I have let him know that I'm available to lend him a helping hand should he need it.

Pediatric Acupressure

As a parent, you naturally want to maximize your child's immune system. I've provided you with a template for using acupressure to do just that. FYI, almost all of the acupoints that you've learned can apply when treating your child, albeit with a far gentler hand (or you may use a warm Tiger Warmer) than you might when working on yourself. The trick, of course, is to be doubly attentive to them.

As you gently massage your baby using circular movement with one finger, be attentive to their reaction. If you sense that they're not clearly enjoying it, stop and wait a while. Then try again, but more gently. If they like the way it feels (you'll know it), massage them for several minutes nightly. Several of the points used in Meridian Tapping coincide with the Chinese acupoints, from which they were borrowed:

DU20=Top of Head Point.

GB1=Side of Head point

DU26=Under Nose point

To strengthen your child's immune system

1) Massage their spinal column from DU14 down to Ming Men, an area on the back between the kidneys and two inches below the navel. For sleep-deprived babies, Ming Men is a wonderfully soothing zone, and a powerful point in Chinese medicine. First focus on calming your mind with your breathing. Once you become calm, simply place your hand on Ming Men, and experience your child slowly nodding out.

2) Massage the area around the navel. If you're doing it right, your baby's face will have a pleased expression. If your child is constipated or has diarrhea, use the points around the belly, primarily CV12 and CV6, as well as ST36). and SP6, and DU1. If they are having diarrhea add DU20.

If you suspect asthma or other breathing issues massage CV17, ST36 and 1.5 inches lateral to DU14.

If they are not responsive to those points, gently massage DU 26.

If they're having difficulty sleeping, gently massage KI1.

As always, when your child is unwell, these treatments are not a substitute for going to a doctor.

Anterior View: **Posterior View:**

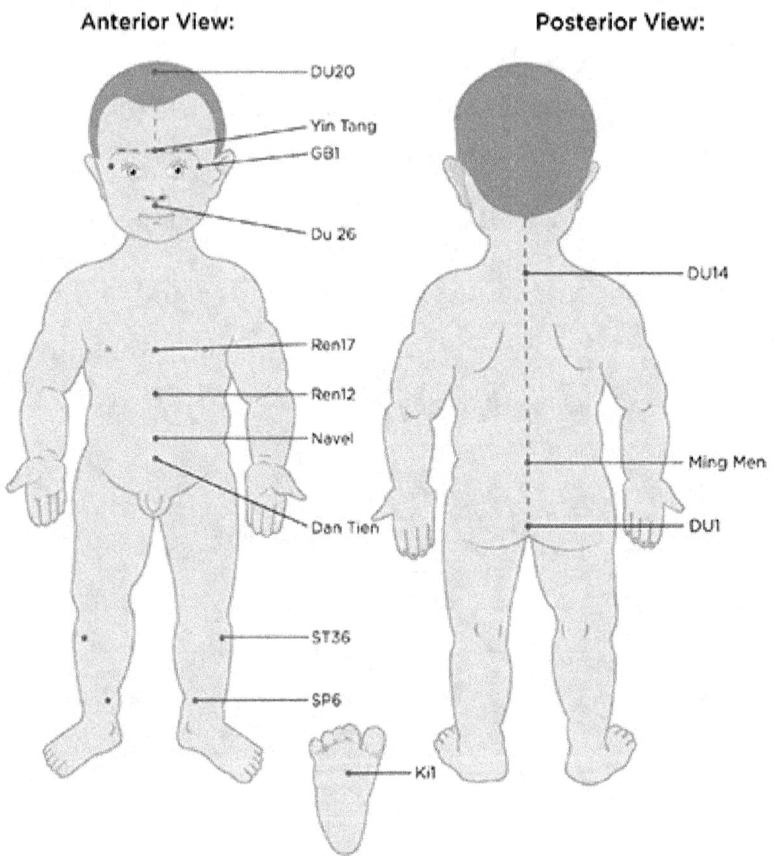

PART III

Journey to the Center

"All healing is an act of Self-Liberation."

– Jeanette Amlie

The Deeper Trek

Perhaps you've been doing the work. Your sleep has improved, along with your overall health. As a result, you're now curious to explore this work on a deeper level. We may think of guided visualization and Neuro-Linguistic Programming as "short-form meditation". The long form is quite simply, "meditation". I've included two forms here: The Inner Smile and The Microcosmic Orbit. They are both part of Qi Gong, and while they dovetail into one another, they also work as standalone modalities.

Meditation

There is a saying that applies: "Don't just do something, stand there." This deep and wide system for enriching our inner world has enough styles and philosophical underpinnings to fit anyone's tastes. For those who may consider meditation to be a club from which they are excluded, know this: all that's required for membership is the curiosity to explore our internal wiring in a safe manner.

Over the years I've practiced two kinds of meditation (and there are many, many forms): Buddha style and Taoist form. In Buddha style, one repeats a word or phrase, or mentally follows the breath.

After a long day, Buddha style works beautifully to offload the psychic junk that has seeped in from all around. And it does far more than that.

A goal of the Taoist form is often to calm the mind, while building internal Qi that may then be accessed as needed to help heal the body. The following exercises are part of the Taoist tradition.

Inner Smile Part I

You can listen to Inner Smile at rewiredforsleep.com/the-deeper-levels.

The goal of this guided meditation seems implausibly grand: to expand the mind to the furthest reaches of the universe and then shrink it down into your umbilicus. And yet, anyone can do it.

Sit straight up in a chair, with your hands on your lap. There's no time limit. As you become comfortable with the sequence, you'll run through it in a minute or two. Read the exercise through until you've memorized it. As an FYI, Inner Smile doesn't work precisely on sleep so much as reduce stress, anxiety, and even a tendency toward depression.

Massage Yintang and Kidney 1 twenty-four times, first clockwise and then counter-clockwise. Close your eyes and take three long, deep breaths into your abdomen. Exhale slowly. Then, smile. See yourself smiling. Take another long, slow, deep breath in, and slowly exhale.

Send the Smile up to Yintang. Place your attention there and visualize yourself exhaling from Yintang. The area may begin to feel warm. Keep your awareness there and notice any feeling that may arise. Take a deep breath in, and as you do so, imagine that you can move the Smile down your throat, out to your arms and down your torso, your back and buttocks, down your thighs and calves, all the way to your toes. Take another deep breath in, and then breathe out. Let the Smile encompass your entire body. Imagine that your Smile is now a large bubble, and you are comfortably inside of it. Notice its color. Is it purple, or white, or clear, or another color? This is your protective bubble; use it anytime you feel invaded by people or situations that are stressful.

Imagine you see, or feel, the Smile bubble expanding, until it encompasses the room. Use your breath, so that when you exhale, you're making the surrounding bubble larger. This sort of visualization exercise might not come naturally to you, and you do not need to do this perfectly.

Keep expanding the Smile, giving each area roughly ten seconds. Don't overthink it. Let your Smile encompass your home; then your street and expanding it to take in your town or city. Then your state. Allow your imagination to run free and even go wider now; expand your smile to encompass your country, the continent, the entire world. Expanding even more now, include the solar system. Then the galaxy. Let your awareness embrace the universe.

Now reverse the process. See, or feel, the Smile enfold the galaxy; then the solar system, and then earth. Shrink the bubble further so it surrounds the continent, your state, your city, your street, and now, your building. Finally, let the bubble encircle your room, and then let it surround your body. As it gets smaller yet, imagine it's the size and shape of a white pearl. You've now got the universe in a small, white pearl. Use your mind to place it 1 1/2 inches below, and behind, your umbilicus. You have just completed the Inner Smile. You've also gathered a source of energy and placed it below your navel. With some practice, you'll be able to access it at will.

This next exercise has two steps. In the first one, you're introduced to the "Microcosmic Orbit." This entails opening two separate energy channels, a front channel and a back one. You connect them, as shown in the illustration below using your imagination. Together, they form a sort of energetic wheel, which you may then use for therapeutic purposes to move energy to other parts of your body.

Microcosmic Orbit

If possible, take a class in Qi Gong. It's my hope that after reading this small piece, you'll want to explore this amazing system more fully. Also, it helps to do the Inner Smile first, but it's not a prerequisite.

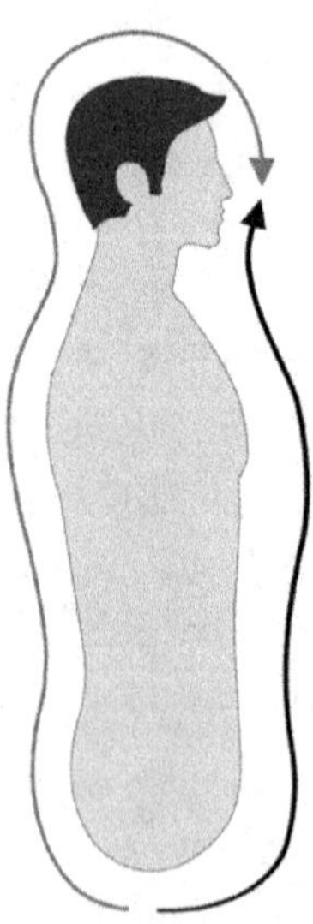

1. Create a relaxed, quiet environment. Wear loose-fitting clothing, especially around your middle. Take off your shoes. Sit with your butt at the edge of a chair. Your back should be straight, and you should be facing straight ahead, with eyes closed. Vigorously rub your hands together for one minute, as if you're washing them with a bar of soap, and massage PC8 in particular.

2. Collect saliva in your mouth for roughly one minute.

3. Massage Yintang and then Kidney 1 twenty-four times in each direction. Imagine that you're breathing through the soles of your feet.

4. Place your palms on your belly, one atop the other. Rotate them around your umbilical area twenty-four times (men clockwise and women counter-clockwise) and imagine that your belly is getting warm.

5. Visualize two clear vessels in your body. One of them begins at your perineum, the dime-sized area between your anus and your genitals and runs up your front of you, along your center, past your belly, chest, and throat, and up to the roof of your mouth. Imagine that the other vessel starts at your anus and travels up your spine, over the top of your head and down to the roof of your mouth. (See the above diagram.)

6. See, or feel, the two vessels meeting at your hard palate, Once you have connected the front and back vessels,

imagine they're a single, energetic "wheel" and it's rotating through you as if it were an orbit going through you. This image might come quickly, or it might take time. Everyone is different. Don't worry that you might not be doing it right. The trick is to keep doing it until it feels like part of you.

7. Imagine that the saliva in your mouth is honey and has healing properties. Swallow it, and feel the healing energy as it goes down your throat, your esophagus. See it going down into your stomach, small intestine, large intestine, and out to your bloodstream to bring nourishment to your body.

Inner Smile II

You can connect the Inner Smile to Microcosmic Orbit. With Inner Smile, you expanded your awareness out to the universe then shrank the universe to a small white pearl an inch and a half below your navel. Apply light pressure and breathe into it. Use your breath like a bellows to pump heat into the white pearl.

Close your eyes and imagine that you can smile into them. Feel a warm smile shine in through your eyes. Now, place your focus on your navel and see, or feel, the white pearl beneath it. Imagine the pearl is circulating energy first in one direction then in the other direction, twenty-four times.

Day 1: Spend five minutes seated. Imagine the orbit spinning in both directions

Day 3: Increase to six minutes

Day 5: Repeat

Day 9: 7 minutes

Day 12: Repeat

Day 14: 8 minutes

Day 16: Repeat

Day 18: 9 minutes

Day 20: 10 minutes

Continue to do this, till you're doing it for twenty minutes, twice a day.

You can listen to a recording of Microcosmic Orbit at rewiredforsleep.com/the-deeper-levels.

Autogenic Training, Part II

Autogenic Training and Progressive Muscle Relaxation are less similar to one another than they might first appear. AT is a form of self-hypnosis as well as a tool for relaxation. As you do AT, you're expanding the ability of your mind to control your body. PMR is a powerful tool for muscle relaxation. Experiment with both methods to see which one you prefer or alternate between them, as desired.

With your eyes closed, focus on your right arm and say to yourself, aloud or silently, "My right arm is heavy and warm. My right arm is heavy and warm." Imagine that arm is both heavy and warm. And then, say it to yourself, "My right arm is warm and heavy."

Focus on the left hand. "My left hand is heavy and warm; my left hand is heavy and warm."

Next, focus on your neck and shoulders, and say to yourself, "My neck and shoulders are heavy, heavy, heavy …"

Now focus on your heart rate and say to yourself: "My heart rate is calm and regular. My heart rate is calm and regular." Repeat to yourself, "My heart rate is calm and regular."

Now, as you focus on your left leg, say to yourself, "My left leg is heavy and warm."

Now, as you notice how you feel, say: "My legs are heavy and warm."

Now move your awareness to your stomach. "My solar plexus is warm and comfortable."

Now notice the forehead and the feeling of coolness on the forehead. And say to yourself, "My forehead is cool ..." and repeat that several times to yourself.

Count from one to five and reorient back into the room.

The 7-Day Neuroplasticity Challenge

Every species thrives on the habitual. When we repeat actions that are familiar to us, we keep stress at bay and enhance our chances of survival. Inversely, when we engage in new activities that have positive consequences, that also has the effect of upping our game and thus raising our chances of survival.

The 7-Day Neuroplasticity Challenge makes a game of exploring the "new." Go the full week if possible. We all have repetitive patterns of behavior, some of which we continue doing even when they no longer serve us. If that sounds like something you might do, it's not an opportunity to beat yourself up. If anything, it's an open door to locating patterns that support you in the most vibrant way possible. The goal isn't to change who you are, but to give you options. One such option might include sleeping fully through the night.

If after doing this exercise you feel more alive than you usually do, and you want more of that, repeat the 7-Day Neuroplasticity Challenge for another week. If not, it probably means you prefer the known ... and welcome to the club. Either way, the Challenge is a low-impact way to assess the limits of your comfort zones, and your flexibility. In case you hadn't noticed it, flexibility is a survival tool in our post-modern world, and you want more of it.

Change Things Up (a V-A-K Trifecta)

If you normally wear a T-shirt to bed, wear pajamas instead. If you're typically eight minutes late to work, show up six minutes early. If you don't speak up at work, contribute in every meeting you can. If you always eat with the veggies on the left part of your plate, place them on the right side. If you are angry with your partner and pick at them in small, passive-aggressive ways, give them a hug, a kiss, and walk away knowing you've messed with their mind — and, more importantly, yours as well.

Why would you bother doing any of this? In part, we want to remind our subconscious that we're never stuck in a state that doesn't benefit us; that in fact, we're always available for rewiring should we want it. You can even imagine that you're seven years old, and this is a game that you've created. Change the pattern anytime you want to. I'd suggest you plan out the changes in your sleep journal so you can refer to them daily. Here are a few suggestions:

Play with the way you comb your hair. Nothing too radical, just a bit ... different. Make this a game to see who notices, and who doesn't. Exercise a bit more, or differently, by adding five minutes to one part of your workout. If you love sugar, substitute fruit. Try drinking tea on the weekend instead of coffee, or even make yourself a Turmeric-Cola!

Behavior: Smile at the person you normally grunt at and notice their response. Walk twice around the block after work to release negative build-up from the job. Massage your feet, or even those of a loved one (notice how they respond to your Ninja skills in gently locating their "ouchy" points). Give yourself a hug, or at least a smile, when looking in the mirror.

Most important, keep the process fun. That too, is a survival tool in our post-mod world.

Meridian Tapping II: Other Voices, Other Modules

We've explored the idea of using Meridian Tapping in order to relieve unwanted grief, and for anger. The following examples show you how you may also use it to address a variety of other issues including Anxiety, Drug Detoxification, Hot Flashes, and Pain. Familiarize yourself with the arcs that I've laid out, that way you may create your own arc as needed. Once you've done the exercise a few times you'll find it all becomes much, much easier.

Anxiety

(Karate point) "Even though I often feel anxiety, I completely and totally accept myself."

(Inner brow) "Feel anxiety."

(Outer eye) "Accept."

(Under eye) "Letting go."

(Below nose) "Accept."

(Below mouth) "Relax instead."

(Collarbone) "I'm only human."

(Under arm) "Sometimes love and accept."

(Top of head) "Accept and love myself."

Round 2

(K) "Anxiety."

(I) "Anxiety."

(O) "Sometimes feel anxiety, sometimes no."

(UE) "I'm only human."

(UN) "Anxiety comes and goes."

(UM) "Totally and completely accept myself."

Drug Detoxification:

(Karate Chop) "Even though my body wants_______, I totally and completely accept myself."

(Eyebrow) "Body wants. Totally accept."

(Side of eye) "Body wants to let go of drugs."

(Under nose) "Letting go of drugs. Accept myself."

(Chin) "Slowly letting go, accept myself."

(Collarbone) "Only human, love and accept myself."

(Under arm) "Body letting go of toxins."

(Top of head) "Totally love and accept myself."

Hot Flashes

Round 1

(K) "Even though I have these _____ (annoying, exhausting, tiring) hot flashes, I truly and completely accept myself."

(EB) "Hot Flashes. I want them to STOP now."

(Temple) "Heat, accept myself."

(Below nose) "Release heat; truly love and accept myself."

(Chin) "Let go of anger, accept myself."

(Collarbone) "Release fear, love myself."

(Top of Head) "Love myself. Totally accept."

Round 2

(K) (subtly shifting time frame) "Even though I've been suffering from these night sweats, I truly and completely love and accept them."

(EB) "Normal phase of life, and I love and accept myself."

(Temple) "I just want them to STOP."

(Below nose) (allowing frustration through and creating a shift in muscle memory)

"Only human, letting go of night sweats." (Wholly acceptable to continue with anger if it feels appropriate, but then downshifting to a calmer, more self-caring state.)

(Chin) "Cool as a cucumber, love myself. Screw Night Sweats."

(Collarbone) "Fully and totally accept and love myself."

(Top of head) "Only human, totally accept myself. I'm okay."

Tapping on Pain

Meridian Tapping can help ease pain and discomfort.

1. Focus on the location and intensity of the pain, and rate it on the 1-10 scale, with 10 being intense pain.

2. If the pain is one-sided, tap TW3 twenty-four times using two fingers of the opposite hand, followed by tapping Karate Chop point.

3. If the discomfort is not one-sided, tap either side.

4. Still focusing on the pain, tap both collarbone points (KI27) five times.

5. Rate the pain.

If there's still discomfort, tap and say:

(K) "Even though there's___(back) pain, I totally and completely accept myself."

(Eyebrow point) "Back Pain."

(T) "Back is uncomfortable."

(UE) "Totally accept."

(UN) "Discomfort at back."

(Ch) "I'm only human. Self-accept."

(CB) "Back's not so bad."

(UA) "Getting better."

(TH) "I deserve to be pain free. Feel fine ..."

Round 2:

(K) "Had back pain."

(EB) "Accept myself."

(OE) "Love myself totally."

(UE) "Old discomfort, letting go."

(UN) "Noticing it's disappearing."

(Ch) "Curious about old discomfort ..."

(CB) "Back okay."

(UA) "Accept, knee feels good."

(TH) "Accept myself."

When you've finished the round, rate the level of discomfort. Typically, it will take several rounds before the discomfort is lessened.

Guided Meditation: Your Special Place

These guided meditations are available for listening at https://rewiredforsleep.com/guided-meditations. I've included a shortened written version of each one so you may record your voice. It may differ from the recorded one. Ideally, begin your session with abdominal breathing while gently massaging a calming acupoint. Continue with Progressive Muscle Relaxation, or Autogenic Training, and then the Staircase. If you are still awake, choose from:

The Beach

The Garden Path

Honduran Rainforest (Heart-Centered Meditation)

The Lake

Recordings of all these meditations can be found at https://rewiredforsleep.com/guided-meditations.

The Beach

See yourself on a beach, a sparkling, turquoise blue sea before you. It's a perfect summer's day, neither too warm nor too cool. You feel the sand beneath your toes, a cool breeze flowing through your hair. You smell the sea air, hear the soft cooing of gulls above you. The gentle rippling tide comes in, and it goes out. Out on the calm blue sea, you see sailboats bobbing up and down, as waves roll in and go out. You walk to the water's edge and dip your toes in. The water is refreshing, and you decide to wade in a bit deeper. You feel so relaxed, so calm, calmer than you've felt in a long, long time. You inhale deeply and relax even more.

Listen to The Beach at https://rewiredforsleep.com/guided-meditations

The Garden Path

You're walking along a garden path. It's a perfect day, and a gentle breeze on your skin is neither too warm nor too cool. Feel a sense of calm. To one side you see there are flowers; you hear the soothing sound of birds in the gently swaying trees. You are on a gravel path, and you find the sound of the pebbles underfoot calming. A bench is nearby. It might be made of wood, or stone, or some other material. Perhaps you sit down and close your eyes for a moment, or else you see yourself lying down, in a meadow or in your bed, feeling calm, sleepy. You remember what it was like to sleep easily, the heaviness of your legs, the drowsiness ...

Listen to the Garden Path at https://rewiredforsleep.com/guided-meditations

Honduran Rainforest (Heart-Centered Meditation)

"Take a deep breath in, and with each exhalation imagine a wave of relaxation going through you. Take a second breath in. As you exhale, imagine, feel, or see yourself walking through a cool, mossy rainforest; the sounds of a far-off waterfall are in the background. You take a nice, deep breath in, and the oxygen in your lungs feels so clean, opening your lungs even more now. Perhaps you feel the ground mossy beneath your feet, sponge-like but firm; You smell the lush, green world all about you, and your fingers graze a beautiful orchid. You see a small wood bridge, and you test it first and, finding it's sturdy, you walk across to the other side to an even more lush forest.

Imagine you can bring your mind to your heart; imagine breathing energy through your heart ... there is a stillness in the rainforest, as there is in your heart. Some people envision breath moving in, and out as they breathe. Imagine breathing the silence of the rainforest into your heart, bringing calming energy to every cell, every muscle in your body, healing energy, so breathe in, and out ... You come to a calm river. You could sit there if you wish, and just watch it flow by. You notice there's a boat with a paddle in it nearby. You pul the boat in the water and slowly begin rowing across the river.

Place your hand to your heart to keep your awareness there, as you breathe normally and naturally ... When your mind wanders, as it almost always will, bring it back to your heart, and breathe ...

in less than a minute, you'll begin to feel that shift, as you breathe in, and out. Getting more, and more relaxed … and then your mind wanders, and you can bring it back to your heart. You cross the river onto land, pulling the boat up onto the sand behind you.

You walk up a hill across an old, worn path and see chimney smoke rising from a white cottage. You open the old door and find your favorite meal just waiting for you. As you eat it, you find yourself becoming sleepy, and perhaps you are even deeper relaxed, now. Letting go. The bed is nearby, and you find yourself lying down … breathing in, and out. Letting go. Now.

Listen to Honduran Rainforest on at https://rewiredforsleep.com/guided-meditations

The Lake

You're rowing a boat across a sparkling lake, the sound of gentle waves splashes against the oars; your arms move forward and back at regular intervals, as the sound of the oars breaking the water creates a rhythm all its own. You feel your breath, constant and steady, your back and legs. You're nearing a calm beach at sunset. Let a feeling of calm filter through you as you see, hear and feel yourself there. Breathing purposefully, say to yourself, I deserve calm now.

You see a beach umbrella, and a beach chair under it. Your favorite drink, cool and refreshing, is waiting for you. You leave the boat, walk across warm sand to the umbrella and sit in the beach chair. You pick up the drink and taste it, taking a long, refreshing sip. You close your eyes and feel yourself drifting away, past all of your thoughts, to a calm place.

Listen to The Lake at https://rewiredforsleep.com/guided-meditations

The 28-Day Insomnia Repair Program

Suggested tools:

Tweezers with a rounded edge

Ear seeds

Tiger Warmer, moxa sticks

Herbs: hops), passionflower) and Valerian)

Hopefully you've been writing in your sleep journal and doing the exercises; as a result, they've made a difference and you're sleeping through the night. It's also possible that you're confused about how to begin. It's for that reason that I created the 28 Day Insomnia Repair Program, both in print and online. If you haven't already done so, go to rewiredforsleep.com, and activate your Rewired Sanctuary membership to access the Program (your activation code is at the end of the book just before the Index). It's rich with guided meditations and contains many of the exercises found here. You'll find it's much easier to do the 28 Day program on a daily basis with the help of this online resource. And consistency is the magic sauce of this program. Let's begin with the modules we've created.

Remember, always breathe evenly and relax your muscles to create fertile soil for sleep. Using your journal, home in on what worked for you. If you loved the Betty E. Self-trance, forget the Staircase, or vice versa. If anxiety and pain is hindering your sleep, focus on them. If CBD oil worked better than St. John's Wort), stick with what worked. You've got all the tools you'll need. Use them.

A Couple of Quick and Dirty Repair Methods

Panic attack: Four-Step Trauma Intervention (FSTI), Butterfly Hug, Auricular Trauma Protocol

Digestive issues: Massage or Tiger Warmer on ST36, CV12, Digestive Protocol, Curing Pills (see Rewiredforsleep.com/the-rewired-shop/

Muscular pain: Desensitize Touch Protocol, Po Sum On Oil, Auricular Pain points

Prior to starting out:

1. Start a sleep journal

2. Do the V-A-K sensor (you can find a recording at rewiredforsleep.com/the-deeper-levels or a transcript in Chapter 1) to determine which "type" you are predominantly.

Week One: This is the set-up week (Preparing for the Trek)

Day 1

- Practice Abdominal Breathing for three minutes. As you do so ....

- Massage Anmian, then Yintang, twenty-four times in each direction.

- Read bedroom improvements (Sleep Hygiene). Take three sleep-related actions and note them in your Sleep Journal

- Take notes in your sleep journal as to how you feel about undertaking this journey.

Day 2

Morning:

- Note your average sleep time (number of hours per night)

- Note your average time in bed (number of hours per night)

Evening:

- Massage Anmian and Yintang 24 times in each direction while taking deep breaths.

- Do Five, Five and Five Exercise. Note which part of it seemed most helpful.

- If you are experiencing anxiety, do Reverse Spin

- If you like, do Remake Your Day.

- Listen to Sleep Now on rewiredforsleep.com

Day 3

- Notice hours spent sleeping________ Hours spent in bed________

- Do abdominal breathing for five minutes

- Listen to Autogenic Training

- If there is a punitive voice in your mind, do Move the Voice.

Day 4

- Notice whether what you eat serves your goals, and adjust your diet as needed.

- Be aware of the words you use regarding sleep (see Power of Words).

- Write an affirmation around sleep or rest and make that your sleep mantra.

- Do Autogenic Training or Progressive Muscle Relaxation (5-10 minutes)

Day 5

- If your mind is overactive, do Reverse Spin. Panicky? Use FSTI during the day.

- Progressive Muscle Relaxation. This exercise is most effective when done at night.

- Locate Auricular Insomnia protocol. Press all of the points with a Q-Tip.

Day 6

- Notice hours spent sleeping_______ Hours spent in bed________

- Turn off the cell phone 20 minutes before coming home.

- Take off your "work coat" and hang it up for the evening.

- Use a Q-tip to gently stimulate three auricular points.

Day 7 – Review the Week

- Practice the Anti-Anxiety Anchor five times today and tomorrow.

- At night, stimulate PC6), Yintang and Hrt7

- Listen to Autogenic Training Parts 1 and 2 Reverse Spin

- Review the week; how's it going for you so far?

How many sleep-positive actions did you take on your behalf this week? ________

If you are falling behind, 1) be gentle with yourself and 2) get back on track.

Acknowledge that 'I'm only human', and you're just where you need to be.

Week Two: Detox, Relax, Recharge

Day 8

- Practice Six Healing Sounds (ten minutes). Home in on those that most resonate for you.

- Herbs: make a tea of hops, passionflower and Valerian. Drink nightly.

- Purchase a Tiger Warmer and moxa sticks (rewiredforsleep.com)

- At night, Acknowledge the Voice (Chapter 10)

Day 9

- Listen to Sleep Now or Honduran Rainforest recording

- Reread the Meridian Tapping section and use it on your issue (5 minutes)

- Use "sleep positive" words when talking about sleep (I've experienced sleep issues...)

- If you tend to wake at night, use Short Form Meridian Tapping.

Day 10 - Detox 3:

- At night massage Under 3rd Toe, LV3 and KI6 twelve times in each direction

- Listen to the Staircase; go to Your "Safe Place", describe your Sleep Room.

Day 11

- Do Six Healing Sounds, homing in on the ones that sound best to you.

- At night, massage Yintang, Heart 7 & Kidney 1 twelve times in each direction

- Go over the short form Meridian Tapping points for several minutes.

- Descend the Staircase to Your Special Place. Enter your Sleep Room.

- Listen to Inner Smile

- Notice what you're eating, and affirm that you'll adjust as necessary.

Day 12

- Do at least one, and preferably all, of the following:

- Stimulate sleep points using acupressure or a Tiger Warmer

- Consider amino acid supplements: if hyper, 5-HTP or GABA.

- Do Remake Your Day, Move the Voice or Reverse Spin

- The Staircase, Safe Place. (Note reactions in Sleep Journal)

Day 13

- If you have purchased an essential oil, use it sparingly on Ki1, Yintang and Ht7)

- If you find yourself thinking about past mistakes, Remake Your Day

- Write one or two Affirmations; do Betty E. Self-Hypnosis.

- Progressive Muscle Relaxation is an option.

Day 14 – Review the week

- Rest or repeat what most resonated (your choice)

- Progressive Muscle Relaxation

- Listen to a recording of your choice—something you haven't previously listened to:

- Guided Meditations

- Music for deeper Relaxation

Week Three: Quick Change Artist, or the 7-Day Challenge

Day 15

- Begin the Neuroplasticity Challenge for one full week (found in the Extra Mile 1.5).

- At night, do the 5, 5 and 5 exercise. Note any images that come to you.

- Meridian Tap on your issue, or do the shortened version for sleep.

- Use Ear points for insomnia: Leave ear seeds in the ears.

- Purchase either an herb, herbal formula or a supplement. (If you are unsure as to which one, consider Valerian and/or Melatonin. 5-HTP is also an option.

Day 16

- 7-Day Neuroplasticity Challenge (day 2)

- 5, 5 and 5, or:

- Write down an affirmation and use Betty E Self Hypnosis,

- Purchase the ingredients for Turmeri-Cola

Day 17

- Day 3 of your Neuroplasticity Challenge

- Short form Meridian Tap if you wake up at night.

- Make Turmeri-Cola. Experiment with a gentle sleep-positive herb of your choice

- Look over your Sleep Journal and then do the Five, Five and Five exercise.

Day 18

- 7-Day Neuroplasticity Challenge (day 4)

- Notice your responses to doing the 7-Day Challenge. Write down your impressions

- Have you tried that Turmeri-Cola yet?

Day 19

- 7-Day Challenge (Day 5)

- If your day was uneven, or stressful, de-stress with Remake Your Day

- Six Healing Sounds (Focus on one or two that you most resonate with).

- Listen to Inner Smile

- Continue to decompress, with Progressive Muscle Relaxation or Autogenic Training

Day 20

- 7-Day Neuroplasticity Challenge (Day 6). Keep going, there are just 2 more days to go!

- Record your impressions of the 7-Day Challenge in your Sleep Journal

- Do all Six Healing Sounds, and notice if there's a sound you don't resonate with.

- Use your Tiger Warmer on points that are your biggest barriers to sleep.

- Review Chapter 7, The Case for the Elastic Brain. Write affirmations in your sleep journal and say them aloud to yourself in a mirror for five full minutes. No cheating.

- Practice your new ability to calm your nervous system, with Autogenic Training followed by the Staircase.

- As an alternative, listen to a Guided Meditation to your Safe Place (Beach, Rainforest, etc.)

Day 21

- 7-Day Neuroplasticity Challenge (day 7—last day!)

- Which part of the 7-Day Challenge would you keep doing as a form of self-expansion?

- Create more affirmations, and let them percolate in your mind awhile, as you do the:

- Betty E. Self-Trance. Affirm beforehand how you want to feel afterward.

- Do Inner Smile, especially if you're experiencing sadness/depression.

- Continue with herbs/supplements, and don't be afraid to change them up.

Week Four: Magical Mystery Microcosmic Orbit...

Day 22

- Tiger Warmer on Hrt7, Ki6) and KI1

- Practice Six Healing Sounds

- When anxiety arises, use any of the tools available to you. Reverse Spin is an option.

- If you've experienced PTSD, you can use the Four-Step-Trauma Intervention

- If you're experiencing unruly thoughts that won't go away, use Move the Voice,

- To settle your brain further, use Staircase to your Safe Space (Beach, Rainforest, etc.)

Day 23

- Inner smile and/or Microcosmic Orbit > Inner Smile 2.

- Acupressure/Tiger warmer on relevant ear points.

- Listen to the Guided Meditation of your choice to find your Special Place (Honduran/Lake/Beach etc.)

Day 24

- Take a bit of time to do Inner Smile, and the Microcosmic Orbit.

- Journal on your dreams. Imagine that every character in your dream is a facet of yourself. What might that mean for you?

- Before sleeping, listen to the Staircase, and proceed to a safe place/guided meditation (Beach, Lake, etc.)

Prepare to Fly Solo!

For the last four days (and you may continue to do this work for as long as you like), fly solo using whatever tools most helped you. Repeat what worked or try new methods. This is your guideline, make it specific to your needs.

Day 25

- Magnolia bark (Hou Po)

- Do the Five, Five and Five Exercise, then listen to the Garden Meditation. It rocks.

- Review your Sleep Journal and choose one or two other actions

Day 26

- Listen to the Lake meditation

- Acupressure or Tiger Warmer on three points

- Your choice of self-hypnosis exercise: Betty E or the Staircase

Day 27

- Listen to Beach meditation

- Your choice: Inner Smile, Microcosmic Orbit and Inner Smile II

- Your choice

Day 28

- Review the herbs and supplements you have tried and score each one for its effectiveness.

- If you are experiencing stress, consider taking Cordyceps.

- Microcosmic Orbit, Inner Smile (and celebrate your progress!)

The 28-Day program is a guideline. You have probably noticed that the Program doesn't include all of the tools that are available to you. It's not because the others are less valuable. In fact, I suggest you go through the book and review them all. Because maintaining your healthy sleep is that important.

There's also this: If I haven't made the point enough, we are each unique, and our timetable for repair is equally so. If you've struggled with sleep for years and aren't suddenly "cured", you're not doing it wrong. Your body (and mind), may need time to get out from the "devil it knows" mode, and into a place of health. Give it time to do so. In the meantime, honor yourself for a job well done.

GOOD NIGHT...

Congratulations. You've made it to the end of the book--and perhaps to the start of your inner trek. As always, consistency is a big plus (and perfection is rare). Dig down into your sleep journal and re-read the techniques, methods, tricks, and exercises that you have highlighted. Find five, four, or even three that resonated for you, and do them until you feel you could teach them to others. Then do them some more.

You may find that, sooner rather than later, you're sleeping better than you have been, feeling better than you have been and, perhaps, experiencing life through new senses. Along the way, you may even find yourself dancing to the subtle rhythms of your inner shaman, as you were always meant to do.

Sweet dreams,

Daniel Reinaldo Bernstein, 2019

Just one last thing, a simple request. Please go to amazon.com, or our website at rewiredforsleep.com if you bought it there, and review this book.

Thank you!

DRB

Glossary of Acupoints and Their Functions

Many of these acupoints are shown on my website at https://rewiredforsleep.com/acupoints.

ST2 (Acupoints:Under Eye point in Tapping): Facial pain, deviation of eye and mouth. Red, itchy eye, twitching of eyelid, facial pain.

ST36.: Gastric pain, vomiting, abdominal distention, diarrhea, constipation, aching of knee joint, cough, dizziness, insomnia.

SP6: Menstrual problems, insomnia from stress/overeating; edema, excessive bleeding during period; emotional disorders.

SP9): abdominal pain, distention, diarrhea, edema, urinary incontinence, dysmenorrhea and knee pain

HT7): Cardiac discomfort; irritability, palpitations, insomnia, mania.

SI3 SI3 (Karate Chop in Tapping): (when a loose fist is made, the point is on the outer edge of the hand, below the knuckle). Pain and rigidity of the neck; sore throat; mania; acute lumbar strain night sweating; pain of the fingers, pain in shoulder and elbow.

UB2 (Eyebrow point in Tapping): Headache, blurring of vision; tearing; swelling and pain of the eye; twitching of eyelids.

KI1: Headache, blurring of vision, dizziness, sore throat, loss of voice, loss of consciousness. Clears the brain, calms the spirit.

KI6): irregular menstruation; retention of urine, constipation; insomnia, sore throat, asthma. Eases genital itching; eases mild dizziness.

KI27 (Collar Bone): Relaxes the chest for chest pain; calms the mind; sedates chronic asthma; Used point for depression and grief. An important point for PTSD and for adrenal fatigue

PC6: Palpitations, stuffy chest, nausea, vomiting, insomnia, irritability; neck pain.

PC8: Cardiac pain, mental disorders, epilepsy, gastritis, vomiting, nausea.

TB3 (Triple Burner 3) : Headache, redness of eyes, deafness; tinnitus; sore throat; low back, shoulder and neck pain. Sciatica, vision issues, dizziness.

GB1 (Side of Eye point): Helps eye problems and headaches behind the eyes; migraine.

GB30: Helps with sciatic pain that is mainly in the buttocks

LI4: Effective for headache, painful jaw, back pain, constipation, allergies, eye issues

LV3: PMS symptoms including breast tenderness/pain, dysmenorrhea. Calming: anger, irritability, insomnia, anxiety; Chest/flank pain; Eye issues: blurred vision, red, swollen painful eyes. Digestive issues: Nausea, vomiting, constipation, diarrhea with undigested food.

DU 20 (Top of Head point): Headache vertigo, tinnitus, mental disorders, depression, prolapse of the rectum and uterus. Sleep disorders.

DU 26 (Under Nose point in Tapping): Mental disorders, epilepsy, infantile convulsion, coma, and swelling of the gums.

Under 3rd-Toe: Point used to reduce high blood pressure, reduces stress, palpitations.

CV12: Abdominal pain, indigestion, vomiting, diarrhea.

CV17: Fullness in the chest and intercostal area; nausea.

CV24 (Chin point in Tapping): Mental disorders and facial problems such as Bell's Palsy, paralysis.

Anmian: Insomnia, vertigo, headache, palpitations, mental disorders.

Yintang: Headache, frontal headache, insomnia, anxiety, mental confusion.

Shimien (bottom of foot) is a "Sleep Point." Acupoints by Repair Function:

Tip: You can find diagrams showing all these Acupoint sets arranged in galleries on RewiredforSleep.com

Insomnia: Anmian, Yintang, Heart 7, Kidney 1, Shimian, Pericardium 8

Anxiety: Pericardium 6), Liver 3, CV17

Digestive Issues: Spleen 6, Kidney 6), Stomach 36, CV12, PC6)

Adrenal Exhaustion: Kidney 27 (collarbone point) Kidney 6), Kidney 1

Depression: DU20, Heart 7, Pericardium 6), CV17

Physical Discomfort: Stomach 36, Triple Warmer 3

Stress: CV17, Heart 7), Pericardium 6, Liver 3

Herbs:

Turmeric, Magnolia bark, Hops, Lavender, Valerian, Siberian Ginseng, Cordyceps, CBD, Kava, Restore the Spleen Decoction, Black Cohosh, Wild Yam, Chamomile, Po Sum On Oil, Food

Rewired for Sleep

Herbs:

Turmeric, Magnolia bark, Hops, Lavender, Valerian, Siberian Ginseng, Cordyceps, CBD, Kava, Restore the Spleen Decoction, Black Cohosh, Wild Yam, Chamomile, Po Sum On Oil, Food

Bibliography

A Chinese Physician: Wang Ji and the Stone Mountain Case Histories, by Joanna Grant

Auriculotherapy Manual; Terrence D. Oleson, Ph.D.

Awaken Healing Light of the Tao; Mantak & Maneewan Chia.

Awaken Healing Energy Through the Tao, Mantak Chia

Bach Flower Remedies; Philip M. Chancellor

Chasing the Dragon's Tail: Yoshio Manaka, with Kazuko Itaya and Stephen Birch

Chinese Acupuncture (L'Acuponcture Chinoise); George Soulie De Morant

Chinese Natural Cures; Traditional Methods For Remedy and Prevention by Henry C. Lu

Curing Insomnia Naturally with Chinese Medicine; Bob Flaws

Extraordinary Vessels; Kiiko Matsumoto & Stephen Birch

Finding Effective Acupuncture Points; Shudo Denmei.

Four Step Trauma Intervention: Jeannette Amlie

Fundamentals of Chinese Acupuncture; Ellis, Wiseman, Boss

Handbook of Hypnotic Suggestions and Metaphors; Hammond, Corydon.

Hypnosis for Inner Conflict Resolution: Introducing Parts Therapy; Roy Hunter, MS FAPHP

The Insomnia Workbook, Stephanie A, Silberman, PH.D

In Pursuit of Sleep, by David Sheppard.

Kiiko Matsumoto's Clinical Strategies, In the Spirit of Master Nagano Vol. 1 by Kiiko Matsumoto and David Euler

Insights of a Senior Acupuncturist; Miriam Lee

Integrative Hypnosis, Melissa Tiers

Lectures, Dr. Royal Lee

Magnetic Healing and Meditation; Larry Johnson, OMD C.A.

Richard Bandler's Guide to Trance-Formation (Richard Bandler)

Magnet Therapy: Balancing Your Body's Energy Flow for Self-healing; Holger Hannemann

My Voice Will Go with You: The Teaching Tales of Milton Erickson Edited by Sidney Rosen

Outline Guide to Chinese Herbal Patent Medicines in Pill Form; Margaret A. Naeser, Ph.D.

Patterns of the Hypnotic Techniques of Milton H. Erickson M.D.; Richard Bandler & John Grinder

The Craving Cure; Rena Greenberg

The Noonday Demon, An Atlas of Depression; Andrew Solomon.

The Practice of Chinese Medicine Giovanni Maciocia

The Root of Chinese Chi Kung: The Secrets of Chi Kung Training;

Say Goodnight to Insomnia; Gregg D. Jacobs, PH.D.

The Secondary Vessels of Acupuncture: A Detailed Account of their Energies, Meridians and Control Points; Royston Low

Soft-Wired, How the New Science of Brain Plasticity Can Change Your Life. Merzenich, Dr. Michael.

The Taoist Experience, An Anthology; Livia Kohn

Trance-formations; Bandler Richard.

Trancework: An Introduction to the Practice of Clinical Hypnosis; Michael D. Yapko

Tung's Acupuncture; Dr. Chuan-Min Wang

Turtle Tail and Other Tender Mercies; Traditional Chinese Pediatrics, Bob Flaws.

Understanding Sleep and Dreaming; William Moorcroft

www.thesleepdoctor.com (Psychology Today]]

One in 6 American Adults Say They Have Taken Psychiatric Drugs, Report Says - Benedict Carey, NY Times

(P. 38) (More on Sleeping Pills and Older Adults - Paula Span, NY Times)

The Taoist (book on Qi Gong)

(p. 46) Clinical Manual of Oriental Medicine; Lotus Institute of Integrative Medicine

How to Buy Essential Oils - Aromaweb

Worried? You're Not Alone - Roni Caryn Rabin, NY Times

The Brain-Gut Connection - John Hopkins Medicine - Wellness & Prevention

Gut Feelings–the "Second Brain" in Our Gastrointestinal Systems [Excerpt] - Justin Sonnenburg, Erica Sonnenburg, Scientific American

Bell, V.L. 1925. A Glossary of Indicated Remedies and Disease Names and Definitions. Cincinnati: Lloyd Brothers Pharmacists.

Boericke, W. 1927. Materia Medica with Repertory. 9th. Philadelphia: Boericke & Runyon.

Bruneton, J. 1995. Pharmacognosy Phytochemistry Medicinal Plants. Paris: Lavoisier Publishing.

Ellingwood, F. 1983. (1898). American Materia Medica, Therapeutics and Pharmacognosy. Portland: Eclectic Medical Publications.

Digestive Diseases Statistics for the United States - NIH- National Institute of Diabetes and Digestive and Kidney Diseases (NIDDK))

White, Gregory Lee (2013-08-11T00:00:00+00:00). Essential Oils and Aromatherapy: How to Use Essential Oils for Beauty, Health, and Spirituality (Kindle Locations 988-989). White Willow Books. Kindle Edition.

On the myth of chemical imbalance: Advice: The Brain and Depression – Michael Yapko, Psychology Today

Books You May Find Interesting

Chinese Medicine

Between Heaven and Earth

The Web that Has no Weaver

Awaken Healing Light of Tao, Mantak Chia

Hypnotherapy

My Voice Will Go With You: The Teaching Tales of Milton Erickson

Trance-Formation (Richard Bandler)

Hypnotherapy (Dave Elman)

Trancework: An Introduction to the Practice of Clinical Hypnosis (Michael D. Yapko)

About the Author

Daniel Reinaldo Bernstein has been a New York State licensed acupuncturist since 1995 and a practicing medical hypnotist since 2005. He maintains a private practice, Blue Phoenix Wellness, in the city that sometimes sleeps, where he resides with his wife and their assorted furry creatures. He has, on occasion, been known to travel in order to give seminars on achieving restful sleep, even as he continues to mangle the Blues on his Gibson J-50 guitar in the privacy of his home.

THE REWIRED SANCTUARY

Activate your Sanctuary Membership

The Rewired Sanctuary is a members-only online supplement to Rewired for Sleep. It offers an extensive library of resources including a daily interactive version of The 28-Day Insomnia Repair Program, simple tutorials and sleep journal prompts. Perhaps most important, you'll have access to powerful audio recordings for most of the meditations, exercises and guided visualizations mentioned in Rewired for Sleep.

If you purchased your copy of Rewired for Sleep on Amazon you will need to activate your complimentary Rewired Sanctuary Membership on our website in order to access all of the resources, present and future for no extra charge.

You can do this easily by going to this link https://rewiredforsleep.com/product/rewired-sanctuary-membership/ (you can also find the link in the footer on the website, marked "Sanctuary Activation"). You will need to set up a simple account with username and password and proceed as if you are purchasing the membership – but as an owner of Rewired for Sleep you won't pay anything. When you reach the checkout page input the code below where directed:

REWIRE_SANCTUARY_7830220

INDEX

2

28-Day Insomnia Repair Program, The, 223–38
    Week 1, Preparing for the Trek, 224
    Week 2, Detox, Relax, Recharge, 228
    Week 3, Quick Change Artist, or the 7 Day Challenge, 231
    Week 4, Magical Mystery Microcosmic Orbit, 235

A

abdominal distention, 41, 193, 241
Acupoint Diagrams
    Anmian, 5
    CV 12, 193
    CV 17, 173
    DU 20, 173
    Ear points for auricular acupressure. *See* Auriculotherapy
    GB 30, 50
    HT7, 106
    Ki 1, 65
    Ki 27, 115
    Ki 6 and Ki 1, 189
    Li 4, 10
    LV 3, 107
    Meridian Tapping, 35
    Paediatric Acupressure Points, 197
    PC 6, 107

PC 8, 179

Shimian, 161

SP 6, 111

SP6 and SP9, 88

ST36, 41

TW3, 46

Yintang, 29

Acupoints

Acupoints by Repair Function, 243

Anmian, 5, 161, 224, 225, 243

Cardiovascular 12 (CV12) (Zhong Wan, or Central Stomach)., 243

Cardiovascular 17 (CV17), 243

Cardiovascular 24 (CV24) (Chin point in Tapping), 243

CV12 (Zhong Wan, or Central Stomach)., 193, 197, 224, 243

CV17, 169, 172, 192, 197, 243

DU 20, 242, 243

DU 26, 197, 242

Eyebrow point in Tapping, 241

Gall Bladder 1 (GB1), 242

Gallbladder 30 (GB 30), 50, 242

GB1, 196

Heart 7 (HT7, Shenmen, or Spirit Gate), 105, 179, 230, 241, 243

Karate Chop in Tapping, 241

Karate point [SI point], 37, 164, 241

Kidney 1(Ki 1), 65, 179, 189, 197, 204, 207, 229, 230, 241, 243

Kidney 27, 114, 139, 216, 243

Kidney 27 (Ki 27), 242

Kidney 6 (KI6, Zhao Hai, Shining Sea), 189, 235, 241, 243

Large Intestine 4 (LI 4), 242

Large Intestine 4 (LI4), 10, 164

Liver 3 (LV3), 111, 112, 113, 143, 192, 229, 242, 243

Pericardium 6 (PC 6), 242

Pericardium 6 (PC6, Neiguan\Inner Pass), 106, 107, 179, 227, 243

Pericardium 8 (PC 8), 242

Pericardium 8 (PC8), 179, 207

Shimian (Difficulty Sleeping), 161, 243

Side of Eye point in tapping, 242

Spleen 6 (Sp6), 87, 111, 143, 197, 241, 243

Spleen 9 (Sp 9) (Yin Ling Quan, or Yin Mound Spring), 87, 241

Stomach 36 (ST36, Zu San Li or Leg Three Miles), 41, 169, 170, 197, 224, 241, 243

Top of Head point in Tapping, 242

Triple Burner 3 (TB 3), 242

Triple Warmer 3 (TW3), 46, 164

UB2, 241

Under 3rd Toe, 30, 31, 55, 229, 243

Under Eye point in Tapping, 241

Under Nose point in Tapping), 242

Yintang, 29, 31, 55, 161, 192, 204, 207, 224, 225, 227, 229, 230, 243

Acupressure

for Adrenal Repair, 139

for Sleep, 5

Pediatric, 196

baby massage, 196

adaptogen, 30

addiction to pain pills, 191

ADHD, 63, 86, 137

adrenal fatigue, 137, 138, 139, 140, 242

adrenaline, 30, 138

Affirmations, xxviii, 58, 59, 60, 61, 151, 152, 169, 226, 231, 232, 234

ALANON, 134

allergies, 10, 242

American Sleep Association, The, 1

anger, 40, 71, 112, 178, 184, 213, 215, 242

Anti-Anxiety Anchor, 31, 227

anxiety, xix, xx, xxiii, 1, 4, 7, 14, 23, 33, 45, 54, 70, 105, 127, 137, 147, 152, 163, 172, 182, 183, 223, 235

5-HTP, 86

acupoints for, 5, 29, 30, 41, 94, 105, 106, 132, 139, 177, 178, 179, 192, 194, 242, 243

and Adderall, 63

breathing correctly, 24

cause of insomnia, 9

defused by Four Step Trauma Intervention, 192

essential oils, 159, 160

Exercises, 5, 225

GABA, 30

herbs, 120, 121, 185

Inner Smile Exercise, 204

lifestyle triggers, 24

L-Theanine, 86

Magnolia Bark, 30

medication side-effects, 101

medications, 99, 104

meridian tapping, 213

Meridian Tapping, 213

symptom of drug withdrawal, 191

types of

amygdala based, 127, 176, 183

prefrontal cortex based, 127, 131

appetite, 22, 24, 30, 33, 41, 42, 83, 122

artificial light, 11

asthma, xxii, 63, 197, 241, 242

Auriculotherapy, 91, 93, 247

Depression points diagram, 174

Digestive Issues, 7

Digestive Issues points diagram, 187

Drug Involvement points diagram, 194

ear seeds, 93, 174, 186, 232

Ear Seeds diagram, 93

Insomnia points diagram, 94

Musculoskeletal points diagram, 92

Pain points diagram, 182

Stress points diagram, 144

Trauma Protocol points diagram, 177

Autogenic Training, xxviii, 54, 55, 56, 133, 151, 159, 169, 178, 192, 210, 217, 226, 227, 233, 234

B

babies and children, 196

Bell's Palsy, 243

Betty E. Self-Hypnosis Method, The, 151

Between eyebrows in tapping. *See* Yintang

Big Pharma, 104

bilateral stimulation, xxi, 114, 128

blood pressure, 30, 54, 243

blurring of vision, 241

Body-Integrative methods, xxviii

bodywork, xx, xxix

Breathing

    Abdominal, 24, 178, 224

    with V-A-K, 2

    Yogic, xxvii

Butterfly Hug, The, 114, 130, 169, 179, 192, 224

C

Cardiac discomfort, 241

CBD oil, 6, 223

Chia, Mantak, 17

China, 34, 65, 91

Chinese medicine, 17, xxii, 51, 55, 66, 70, 76, 91, 95, 105, 112, 114, 163, 164, 196

Chinese Medicine, xxii, xxvii, 4, 63, 251

Chunyu Yin, xxix

Circadian Rhythm, xxix, 12, 121

claustrophobia, xx

Cognitive Behavioral Therapy, xxvii, 10

Collarbone Point. *See* Acupoints: Kidney 27

coma, 242

constipation, 10, 41, 193, 241, 242

cortisol, 30, 138

Coue, Emile, 59

cough, 241

D

depression, xix, 33, 54, 94, 105, 121, 127, 130, 138, 170, 173, 174, 175, 188, 242

   5-HTP, 86

   acupoints, 177, 194, 242, 243

   essential oils, 159

   Exercises, 235

   healing sounds, 73

   herbs, 120, 123

   Inner Smile Exercise, 204

   medication side effects, 101

detox. *See* Detoxification

Detoxification, 5, 71, 77, 112, 123, 175, 190, 191, 192, 193, 213, 228

Detoxification, meridian tapping, 214

Detoxification, Tools for, 192

diarrhea, 41, 87, 111, 112, 182, 193, 197, 241, 242, 243

dizziness, 29, 41, 111, 241, 242

E

edema, 87, 111, 241

Egypt, 34, 149

emotional disorders, 241

epilepsy, 242

Epsom salts, 7, 13

Erickson, Betty, 151

Erickson, Milton, 17, 150, 251

essential oils, xxviii, 159

Essential Oils

   Bergamot, 159

   Chamomile, 160

   eucalyptus oil, 13

   Jasmine, 160

Lavender, 160

Neroli, 160

Sandalwood, 160

Eye, 10, 242

blurred vision, 242

blurring of vision, 241

deviation of eye and mouth, 241

eyelid,twitching of, 241

headache/migraine behind, 242

headaches/migraine behind, 242

Healing Sound supports eyesight, 71

painful, 241

Red, itchy, 241

red, swollen painful, 242

redness, 242

swelling, 241

tearing, 241

F

fatigue, 120, 137, 160, 191

fibromyalgia, 140, 163, 164

Five, Five, and Five, The, 6, 187, 225

Food

Sleep-Positive Food, 81

Four-Step Trauma Intervention (FSTI), 128, 131, 192, 224

Free and Easy Wanderer, 192

FSTI. *See* Four-Step Trauma Intervention (FSTI)

Fullness in the chest and intercostal area, 243

G

GABA, 230

gastritis, 242

golf, 28

grief, 36, 71, 75, 213, 242

Guided Meditations
    Honduran Rainforest, 218, 219, 220, 228
    Progressive Muscle Relaxation, xxviii, 6, 34, 45, 47, 151, 192, 210, 217,
        226, 231, 233
    The Beach, 217, 218
    The Garden Path, 218
    The Lake, 218, 220
guided visualization, xxvii, 60, 115, 149, 203
gums,swelling of, 242

H

headache, 46, 66, 111, 242, 243
Headache, 101, 241, 242, 243
Herbs, xxviii, xxix, 1, 6, 30, 63, 105, 119, 122, 123, 149, 158, 169, 175, 235,
    238
    Black Cohosh, 189, 244
    California Poppy, 121
    CBD (Cannabidiol), 121
    Chamomile, 120, 122, 123, 244
    Chinese herbal formulas, 119
    Cordyceps Sinensis, 122, 140, 238, 244
    Formulas for Insomnia, 122
    Ginseng, Korean, 30
    Ginseng, Siberian, 30
    Hops, 120, 223
    Kava, 63, 120, 123, 169, 185, 192, 244
    Kava (Piper methysticum), 120
    Magnolia Bark (Hou Po), 30, 169
    oat straw, 121
    Passionflower (Passiflora), 121, 223
    Restore the Spleen Decoction, 185, 244
    Siberian Ginseng, 244
    skullcap, 49, 120
    Sleep-Positive Herbs, 119
    St. John's Wort, 175

St. John's Wort (Hypericum perforate), 121, 223

Turmeric, 123, 244

Turmeri-Cola, 123, 212

Valerian (Valeriana officinalis), 120, 223

Western Herbs, 120

Wild Yam (Dioscorea villos), 189

Hongling, Tao, 71

Hormones

ghrelin, 83

Growth Hormone (GH), 32

leptin, 83

Hypnopuncture, 163

Hypnosis

Betty E. Self-Hypnosis Method, The, 151

Trance, 17, xx, xxix, 34, 129, 130, 147, 148, 149, 150, 151, 152, 163, 223

anchoring, 23, 130

future work, 148

history of, 149

Hypnosis, 150

Neuro-Linguistic Programming, xxvii, 34, 51, 141, 150, 158, 203

post-hypnotic suggestion, 130

I

IBS, xix, 170, 190

Hypnopuncture, 163

indigestion, 193, 243

infantile convulsion, 242

Inner Smile, 71, 203, 204, 205, 206, 208, 230, 233, 235, 236, 237, 238

irritability, 101, 120, 178, 194, 241, 242

acupoints, 106

J

journaling, xxviii

K

kill-off reaction, 77

Kundalini Yoga, 70

L

Lifestyle, 21, 23

Liu Zi Jue, 70

loss of consciousness, 241

loss of voice, 241

M

mania, 241

meditation, xxvii, 32, 70, 115, 134, 179, 182, 203, 204, 236, 237

melatonin, 12, 82, 86, 87, 94

memory lapses, 138

Menstrual Problems, 241

    depression during menopause, 188

    dysmenorrhea, 87, 241, 242

    excessive bleeding during period, 241

    herbs for hot flashes, 189

    Hot Flashes, 189, 190, 213

    Hot Flashes, meridian tapping, 214

    insomnia during menopause, 188, 190

    irregular menstruation, 241

    menopause, 188, 189

    menstrual disorders, 139

    phytoestrogens and menopause, 190

mental confusion, 243

mental disorders, 242, 243

Meridian Tapping, xxviii, 1, 33, 34, 36, 40, 43, 114, 169, 173, 179, 189, 192, 196, 213, 216, 229

    Emotional Freedom Technique (EFT), 34

meridians, 66, 111

Merzenich, Dr Michael, 53, 249

Mesmer, Franz, 150

metabolism, xxx, 123

Microcosmic Orbit, 164, 203, 206, 208, 209, 235, 236, 237, 238

Ming dynasty, xxix

Move the Voice, 6, 26, 169, 171, 226, 230, 235

moxa, 95, 96, 170, 173, 223, 228

muscle weakness, 138

My Friend John/Jane, 5, 158

N

Napping, 11

nausea, 30, 106, 112, 179, 191, 193, 242, 243

nervousness, 94

Neurons, 28, 51

Neuroplasticity, xx, xxvii, 53, 211, 232, 233, 234

Neuroplasticity Challenge, The, 211, 231

neuroscience, xx

Neuroscience, 27

New York City, 3

night sweats, 194, 215

Nogier, Dr Paul, 91

nutrition, xx, xxix, 23

Nutrition

    avocado, 81

    Bananas, 82

    barley, 82

    buckwheat, 82

    butter, 81

    Cherry juice, 82

    coconut oil, 81

    cravings, 83

    Food to Avoid, 83

    green tea, 81

    high antioxidant foods, 81

high glycemic index, 82

high-nutrient fruits, 81

Hunger, 83

Jasmine rice, 82

leafy vegetables, 81

lima beans, 83

Milk, 82

organic and pasture-raised meats, 81

papaya, 83

potassium-rich foods, 83

potatoes, 83, 85

quinoa, 82

sleep-positive food, 1, 31

Sleep-Positive Food, 81

Sweet potatoes (yams), 83

tryptophan, 82

Turkey, 82

yogurt, 82

O

On Caring for the Health of the Mind and Prolonging the Life Span, 71

Ötzi, 63

overeating, 241

P

Pain

abdominal, 87, 241, 243

auriculotherapy for the relief of, 91

back, 242

breast tenderness, 242

cardiac, 242

CBD Oil, 121

chest, 242

elbow, 241

eye, 241

facial, 241

fibromyalgia, 163

fingers, 241

gastric, 41, 241

headache, 242, 243

headache, 242

jaw, 242

knee, 87, 131, 241

knee, 241

low back, 242

lower back, 46

lumbar, acute, 241

migraine, 242

muscular, 224

neck, 241, 242

sciatic, 50, 242

shoulder, 176, 241, 242

Pain and rigidity of the neck, 241

palpitations, 30, 41, 54, 105, 106, 129, 139, 185, 241, 242, 243

Panic attacks, xxi, 127, 130, 224

paralysis, 243

parasympathetic nervous system (PNS), 22

Patient Case Studies

Annabelle, 169, 182

Barbara, 157

Brody, 63

Darrell, 33

David, 21

Dina, 109

Eamon, 3

Edward, 127

Erika, 148

Helene, xix, 169, 170

Jeffrey, 169, 176

Jenna, 131

Luis, 45
Margaret, 169, 188
Michelle, 137
Raymond, 169, 190
Pauli Exclusion Principle, The, 51, 56
Physical Causes of Insomnia. *See also Pain*
abdominal bloating, 30
digestive issues, xxiii, 9, 87, 104, 112
indigestion, 9
PMS, 111
stomach tension, 9
PMS, 111, 112, 242
PMS acupoints, 111
Po Sum On Oil, 49, 224, 244
Polarity, 14
Prefrontal Cortex, 95, 127, 131, 178, 183
pregnancy, 10, 30, 106, 159
Prescription Drugs
Adderall, 63, 67
Ambien, 100, 104, 176, 194
Benzodiazepines, 99, 100, 191
Lunesta, 100
Oxycodone, 191
Seroquel, 175
Sonata, 100
Vicodin, 191, 195
Xanax, 191
zolpidem, 100, 104
Progressive Muscle Relaxation, 47, 227, 231
prolapse of the rectum and uterus, 242
PTSD, 96, 169, 176, 177, 179, 181, 194, 235, 242

Q

Qi, 66, 69, 70, 71, 95, 159, 203, 204
Qi Gong, 69, 70, 159, 163, 203, 206, 249

R

REM sleep, 30, 86, 102, 104

Remake Your Day, 6, 27, 28, 31, 42, 54, 225, 230, 233

Restless Leg Syndrome (RLS), 3

retention of urine, 241

Reverse Spin, xxviii, 1, 140, 144, 169, 183, 225, 227, 230, 235

Rewired Detox Program, The, 195

Rewired Sanctuary, The, xxx, 255

    Activate Membership, 255

Robbins, Tony, 60

S

Sankalpa, 59

sea-sickness

    acupoints, 106

Sex, 14, 137

shaman, 64

shock, 33

shortness of breath, 41

Six Foundation Stones of Self-Esteem, 150

Six Healing Sounds, 1, 70, 71, 159, 192, 228, 229, 233, 234, 235

    Heart/Small Intestine, 73

    Kidneys/Bladder, 76

    Liver/Gallbladder, 71

    Lungs/Large Intestine, 75

    Spleen/Stomach/Pancreas, 74

    Triple Warmer/Pericardium, 77

Sleep Aids, 103, 190

Sleep Disorders

    Circadian Rhythm Sleep Disorder, xxix

    Narcolepsy, xxix

    sleep apnea, 21, 32

    Sleep Paralysis, xxix

    Somnambulism, xxix

Sleep Hygiene, 9, 10, 14, 225
Sleep Journal, 7, 11, 14, 71, 77, 178, 212, 223, 225, 230, 232, 234, 237
Sleep-positive food therapy, xxviii
sore throat, 46, 139, 241, 242
Stages of Sleep, 102, 158
Staircase, The, 115, 130, 151, 169, 178, 217, 229, 230, 234, 235, 236, 237
Stress, xxii, 17, 21, 24, 54, 59, 104, 109, 137, 138, 147, 211
    abdominal breathing, 25
    acupoints for, 241, 243
    adrenal fatigue induced by, 122
    and insomnia, 1
    and Sex, 14
    and unbalanced lifestyle, 18
    barrier to sleep, 9
    Butterfly Hug as antidote, 114
    Cordyceps, 122, 238
    cortisol, 138
    diarrhea, 182
    foods containing Tyramine, 85
    GABA, 30
    gluten intolerance, 84
    Inner Smile Exercise, 204
    Jasmine Essential Oil, 160
    Magnolia Bark, 30
    neurotransmitters, 22
    Passiflora reduces stress-related insomnia, 121
    Remake Your Day Exercise, 233
    Siberian Ginseng increases resistance, 30
    toxins, 112
Supplements, xxviii, 1, 6, 86, 230, 235, 238
    5-HTP, 86, 133, 230, 232
    Amino Acids, 86
    GABA, 30
    Jarrow (brand), 140
    L-Theanine, 63, 86
    magnesium, 6, 82

magnolia bark, 30

Solgar (brand), 140

Vitamin B, 140

Vitamin C, 140

Vitamin D3, 140, 164

sweating, 30, 194, 241

sympathetic nervous system (SNS), 22, 158

T

Taoism, 71

temperature imbalances, 30

Tiger Warmer, 50, 93, 95, 96, 113, 143, 161, 164, 169, 170, 181, 185, 189, 192, 193, 196, 223, 224, 228, 230, 234, 235, 237

tinnitus, 46, 242

trauma, xxi, xxviii, 34, 104, 114, 128, 129, 131, 177, 192, 224, 235

twenty-minute rule, the, 10

Types of Insomnia

Acute, 1, 33

Maintenance, 1, 100, 169, 176

Onset, 1, 100, 169, 182, 183

Paradoxical, 157, 158

Psycho-physiological, 1, 131

Rebound, 1, 45, 101, 191

U

urinary incontinence, 87, 241

V

vaginal dryness, 139

V-A-K, 1, 2, 28, 148, 151, 153, 154, 212

Auditory Sensor, 2, 3

Kinesthetic Sensor, 2, 3

main sensor, 1

V-A-K Sensor, 2, 28

Visual Sensor, 2, 3
V-A-K Sensor Exercise, 224
vertigo, 29, 54, 242, 243
visualization, 78, 205
vomiting, 41, 101, 112, 193, 241, 242, 243

W

Wang Ji, xxix, 247
weight gain, 138
wise women healers, 17, 64
Worry Session, 24

Y

yoga, xxix, 25, 109, 137